Breast Cancer Survivorship Care

A Resource for Nurses

Lillie D. Shockney, RN, BS, MAS

Administrative Director
Johns Hopkins Avon Foundation Comprehensive Breast Center
University Distinguished Service Associate Professor of Breast Cancer
Associate Professor, Departments of Surgery and Gynecology
Johns Hopkins University School of Medicine
Associate Professor
Johns Hopkins University School of Nursing
Baltimore, Maryland

JONES AND BARTLETT PUBLISHERS
Sudbury, Massachusetts
BOSTON TORONTO LONDON SINGAPORE

World Headquarters
Jones and Bartlett Publishers
40 Tall Pine Drive
Sudbury, MA 01776
978-443-5000
info@jbpub.com
www.jbpub.com

Jones and Bartlett Publishers
Canada
6339 Ormindale Way
Mississauga, Ontario L5V 1J2
Canada

Jones and Bartlett Publishers
International
Barb House, Barb Mews
London W6 7PA
United Kingdom

Jones and Bartlett's books and products are available through most bookstores and online booksellers. To contact Jones and Bartlett Publishers directly, call 800-832-0034, fax 978-443-8000, or visit our website, www.jbpub.com.

Substantial discounts on bulk quantities of Jones and Bartlett's publications are available to corporations, professional associations, and other qualified organizations. For details and specific discount information, contact the special sales department at Jones and Bartlett via the above contact information or send an email to specialsales@jbpub.com.

Production Credits
Publisher: Kevin Sullivan
Acquisitions Editor: Emily Ekle
Acquisitions Editor: Amy Sibley
Associate Editor: Patricia Donnelly
Editorial Assistant: Rachel Shuster
Senior Production Editor: Carolyn F. Rogers
Senior Marketing Manager: Barb Bartoszek
V.P., Manufacturing and Inventory Control: Therese Connell
Composition: diacriTech
Cover Design: Scott Moden
Cover Image: © Galina Barskaya/Dreamstime.com
Printing and Binding: Malloy, Inc.
Cover Printing: Malloy, Inc.

Library of Congress Cataloging-in-Publication Data
Breast cancer survivorship care : a resource for nurses / [edited by] Lillie D. Shockney.
p. ; cm.
Includes bibliographical references and index.
ISBN 978-0-7637-8496-6 (pbk.)
1. Breast–Cancer–Nursing. 2. Breast–Cancer–Patients–Long-term care. I. Shockney, Lillie, 1953-
[DNLM: 1. Breast Neoplasms–nursing. 2. Breast Neoplasms–psychology. 3. Nurse-Patient Relations. 4. Survivors–psychology. WY 156 B828 2011]
RC280.B8B68895 2011
616.99'4490231–dc22

2009046935

6048

Printed in the United States of America
13 12 11 10 09 10 9 8 7 6 5 4 3 2 1

Contents

Preface

Breast cancer remains the most common malignancy and one of the most feared diseases in American women. Thanks to advances in screening and therapy, the mortality rate from breast cancer is dropping, and it appears that age-adjusted incidence is also decreasing. Estimates for 2009 from the National Cancer Institute suggest that approximately 192,370 women and 1,910 men will be diagnosed with invasive breast cancer and an estimated 45,000 individuals will receive a diagnosis of in situ cancer. Approximately 40,170 women and 440 men will succumb to the disease, but 85% will survive.

These statistics imply that many primary care, gynecology, and internal medicine physicians and advanced nurse practitio-ners will be involved in the assessment, diagnosis, treatment, and long-term evaluation of such patients. The information written for you in this guide is specific for advance practice nurses and the important role you can provide in serving as the breast cancer survivor healthcare provider.

Breast cancer diagnosis and treatment is a rapidly evolving field. This book is designed to provide succinct information on how to assess and manage breast cancer survivors for long-term follow-up. It includes information about performing a health assessment, when and how to refer a patient for diagnostic breast evaluation if needed, how the patient's breast cancer treatment might affect other medical conditions, and the role of surveillance during and after treatment. It also contains specialized topics such as menopausal management, examination of reconstructed or radiated breasts, and evidence-based follow-up algorithms. Primary care physicians, oncology nurses, advance practice nurses, gynecologists, and other healthcare professionals play an important role in the care and monitoring of breast cancer survivors after treatment is completed, because they are in a position to address the full spectrum of the cancer survivor's health needs. In fact, randomized trials conducted in the United Kingdom and Canada show that survival for patients who have completed their treatment for early breast cancer is equal whether they are followed by their cancer specialist or their primary care provider. Therefore, it is likely that nononcologists will be increasingly engaged in longitudinal care of breast cancer survivors.

This book is divided into sections to make it as easy as possible to find the information you need, whether it is related to survivorship care (addressing long-term side effects, promoting a healthy lifestyle to reduce risk, assessing psychological needs of survivors), basic breast health assessment, breast cancer prevention, and promotion of breast cancer screening for early detection. The authors are members of the Johns Hopkins University School of Medicine faculty and staff who specialize in the assessment, diagnosis, treatment, prevention of breast cancer, and long-term follow-up of breast cancer patients.

Once a patient's treatment is completed, she will be seen less frequently by members of her breast cancer medical team and may be transitioned to you for her long-term care. Our goal for this book is to provide advance practice nurses and their patients with the necessary information to ensure continuity of care, to optimize general health, and to reduce the risk of breast cancer recurrence while promoting and maintaining a good quality of life.

This is an exciting new career path for many nurse practitioners. We hope this information is valuable to preparing you in your role as the healthcare provider managing breast cancer survivors post treatment.

Introduction

A great deal of thought and consideration was given to deciding what information should be contained in this book. The goal was to provide an easy-to-read guide to assist advanced practice nurses in the fields of gynecology, oncology, internal medicine, and primary care in the monitoring and long-term management of breast cancer survivors as well as provide guidance regarding the assessment and care of women with other breast health issues or abnormalities.

Currently 77% of women diagnosed with breast cancer are age 50 or older; however, it is projected that approximately 66% of the new cases diagnosed will occur in women younger than age 65.[1] We have seen and treated a large number of young women at Johns Hopkins in recent years and have certainly seen a growing number of young women entering our breast center doors. No doubt you have seen an increase in the incidence of the disease among your own patients in addition to perhaps their age group getting younger. Breast cancer is no longer considered a disease of older women.

Because of the increased incidence of this disease and the impending shortage of oncology specialists (projected to be a 48% deficit by 2020), the necessity to transition patients away from oncologists (surgeons, medical oncologists, and radiation oncologists) sooner is becoming imperative. As mentioned in the preface of this text, an article in the *Journal of Clinical Oncology* entitled "Randomized Trial of Long-Term Follow-up for Early Stage Breast Cancer—A Comparison of Family Physician vs Specialist Care" confirms that survival is equal for patients, whether followed long-term by their oncologist, gynecologist, or primary care provider.[2] In this specific study, concentrated education was provided to these healthcare professionals before the transition began. It is not realistic to expect nurse practitioners who have not been following breast cancer survivors' long term to automatically have the knowledge to appropriately and confidently follow this unique patient population.

The pressure to do so and the expectations of patients will be high. Though the timing of when a patient may be transitioned to your care may vary by stage of the patient's disease and other clinical and psychological factors, the final outcome will be that these patients will no longer be able to occupy the exam room of oncology specialists who will need to be making room for more newly diagnosed patients. Statistics for 2009 estimate that there will be 192,370 women and 1,910 men diagnosed with invasive breast cancer and more than 45,000 individuals diagnosed with ductal carcinoma in situ (DCIS), the most common type of noninvasive breast cancer. Additionally, approximately 40,170 women and 440 men will have died.[1] With baby boomers now in midlife, these numbers will continue to grow. Primary care providers, advanced practice nurses, gynecologists, and other healthcare professionals will play an increasingly important role in the monitoring and care of breast cancer survivors after treatment is completed. Nurse practitioners may be especially well positioned based on their nursing role in health assessment, health maintenance, and disease prevention, to address the full spectrum of cancer survivor health needs, provided they are empowered with the information they need to confidently manage their patients' long-term follow-up care.

Some healthcare providers may not be familiar with the clinical assessment and diagnostic steps needed to evaluate patients with a breast health problem, or even with the optimum time to refer patients for additional workup at a comprehensive breast center. A delay in the diagnosis of breast cancer remains a leading cause of medical malpractice today.

The information contained in this book is intended to provide the knowledge you need as a nurse practitioner working in women's health, with a specific focus on breast health and breast cancer survivorship. This book contains information targeted toward survivorship care; however, it also contains information related to the types of technology used today for diagnosing breast health problems, both benign and malignant, and the many long-term side effects that your patients may experience, following completion of their treatment and transition to your care. A special focus has been given to addressing the medical needs and psychological well-being of the breast cancer patient after her adjuvant therapy is finished. She will be seeing you more often and seeing her oncology team less frequently, and, in most cases, perhaps not seeing a cancer specialist at all—acknowledging *you* as her breast cancer survivor specialist.

The information, broken down by chapters, includes the diagnostic tools available and when and who should order them, your important role after treatment is completed to help maintain the patient's breast health and overall health and survivorship status, and even information related to assessing the patient and her family for possibly having a genetic predisposition to developing breast cancer. Pharmacogenetics information is provided as well, given that patients can be on a variety of other medications unrelated to their breast cancer treatment that may negatively influence the effectiveness of prescribed cancer treatments, such as hormonal therapy.

Furthermore, you will find evidence-based medicine that supports ways to reduce your patient's long-term side effects related to treatment, for which she will seek your guidance. There is also specific information about the importance of helping patients maintain compliance with their treatment, particularly hormonal therapy that needs to be taken for several years after other treatment has ended. This is also applicable for promoting adherence with cancer screenings and living a healthy lifestyle to reduce future cancer diagnoses.

This book contains a variety of algorithms and charts, as well as a frequently asked questions (FAQ) section at the end of each chapter. These are intended to provide you with a quick reference for specific information that you may need and supporting documentation within the context of the chapter.

As an additional aid for you and your patients, we have provided a resource chapter in the back of this book. It contains a list of credible organizations that provide educational information and support to patients and their families who are journeying through breast cancer treatment and beyond. This information is there for you to share with your patients as you take on the challenge of managing the care of women with breast health problems and care for breast cancer survivors.

Of great importance is the management of your patient's psychological well-being. Transitioning from her oncology team to you for survivorship care can be anxiety provoking. She will be looking to you for advice and needs to feel confident she is in good hands. I hope this information prepares you with the guidance and tools you need to feel expert in breast cancer survivorship management.

Lillie D. Shockney

REFERENCES

1. National Cancer Institute. Breast cancer home page [Web page]. Available at: http://www.cancer.gov/cancertopics/types/breast. Accessed September 25, 2009.
2. Grunfeld E, Levine MN, Julian JA, et al. Randomized trial of long-term follow-up for early-stage breast cancer: a comparison of family physician versus specialist care. *J Clin Oncol.* 2006;24(6):848-855.

About the Editor

Lillie D. Shockney, RN, BS, MAS

Administrative Director, Johns Hopkins Avon Foundation Breast Center; Associate Professor of Surgery and Gynecology, Johns Hopkins University School of Medicine

Mrs. Shockney is a registered nurse with a BS in Health Care Administration from Saint Joseph's College and a master's in Administrative Science from Johns Hopkins University. She has worked at Johns Hopkins since 1983 and has served as the Administrative Director since 1997. As Administrative Director she is responsible for the quality-of-care programs; patient education programs; the survivor volunteer team; community outreach at the local, regional, and national levels; webmaster, and patient advocacy.

Mrs. Shockney has written 12 books and more than 200 articles on breast cancer and is a nationally recognized public speaker on the subject. She serves on the medical advisory board of several national breast cancer organizations and is the cofounder and vice president of a national nonprofit organization called "Mothers Supporting Daughters with Breast Cancer."

She is also the recipient of the Global Business Leadership award, numerous community service awards, was the recipient of the Outstanding Women of America Award, in 1997 was awarded the Distinguished Graduate for Lifetime Achievement Award, and in 1998 received the National Silver Medal Award from the National Consumer Health Information Center. In 1999 she was the recipient of the National Circle of Life Award and the American Cancer Society's Voice of Hope Award; in 2001, she was the recipient of the ACS Lane Adams Award for Excellence in Caring; in 2000, she was selected as an "Unsung Hero" for breast cancer by Pharmacia & Upjohn's 2001 calendar. She also received the 2001 Lane A. Adams Award for Excellence in Caring from the American Cancer Society. In addition, Mrs. Shockney has received the 2002 Faces of Breast Cancer, ACS, and the 2002 Oncology Nursing Society Award for Excellence in Breast Cancer Education awards. In 2003 she was the recipient of the Impact Award from the National Consortium of Breast Centers. She was also the recipient of the Komen Award from the Maryland Affiliate in 2003. In 2004 she was a finalist for the Lance Armstrong Foundation's Spirit of Survivorship award and was selected as one of the Top 100 Women in Maryland for her leadership and community service efforts. Mrs. Shockney was selected by the Komen Foundation, nationally, to receive the 2005 Professor of Survivorship Award. In 2006 she was the recipient of the Spirit of Friends Award from Food & Friends and the Avon Foundation, and also received the Patient of Courage Award from the American Plastic Surgery Society. Mrs. Shockney was the recipient of the 2007 Yoplait Breast Cancer Champion award. She received the 2009 ONS Excellence in Survivor Advocacy Award and, also in

2009, she received the Maryland Daily Record Healthcare Hero—Nursing Excellence Award.

In 2008, the Johns Hopkins Board of Trustees made a decision to appoint her to a chair as a University Distinguished Service Assistant Professor of Breast Cancer. This is the first time in the history of the institution that a hospital nurse has been appointed to a distinguished service designation.

She serves as "Ask an Expert" for several breast cancer Web sites including Yahoo.com and the Johns Hopkins Breast Center's Web site. She chairs the National Consortium of Breast Centers QI Task Force. Mrs. Shockney also holds a faculty appointment as Associate Professor in the Departments of Surgery and Gynecology within the Johns Hopkins University School of Medicine, and is an active clinical researcher with a focus on quality-of-life issues for survivors.

Contributors

Charles Balch, MD
Professor of Surgery and Oncology

Dr. Balch has been a Professor of Surgery and Oncology at Johns Hopkins since 2000. He has been a surgical oncologist for over 30 years, specializing clinically in breast cancer and melanoma. He received his medical degree at Columbia College of Physicians and Surgeons. Dr. Balch was trained in surgery at Duke Medical Center and the University of Alabama at Birmingham. He also completed a fellowship in immunology at Scripps Clinic and Research Foundation.

Dr. Balch has published over 560 scientific articles, book chapters, and abstracts, including numerous scientific articles and book chapters specifically about breast cancer. He was the founding Editor-in-Chief of the journal *Breast Diseases* as well as the founding Editor-in-Chief of *The Annals of Surgical Oncology*. He has held numerous leadership roles including Executive Vice President and CEO of the American Society of Clinical Oncology; President and CEO of the City of Hope National Medical Center; Chief of Surgery and Anesthesiology, Vice President of Hospital and Clinics, and Executive Vice President for Health Affairs at the University of Texas MD Anderson Cancer Center; and Chief of Surgical Oncology, Associate Director and Acting Director of the Comprehensive Cancer Center at the University of Alabama in Birmingham. He also has been President of the Association for Academic Surgery and the Society of Surgical Oncology and Chair of the Commission on Cancer for the American College of Surgeons. Dr. Balch is the recipient of the Society of Surgical Oncology's Heritage Award, 2006.

Nagi F. Khouri, MD
Director, Johns Hopkins Breast Imaging
Associate Professor of Radiology

Dr. Khouri earned his MD degree from the American University of Beirut in 1971. Following his residency training at Johns Hopkins in 1975, he was board certified in radiology and joined the full-time faculty as a chest radiologist from 1976 to 1986, where he was the head of that section. His clinical interests and research focused on lung cancer, computer tomography (CT) of the pulmonary nodule, and percutaneous lung biopsies. Since 1986, he has focused all of his efforts on the field of Breast Imaging and Intervention, first at the Diagnostic Breast Center of Cross Keys and later as the Director of Breast Imaging at Johns Hopkins at Green Spring-Station. His major areas of interest are breast imaging and intervention with a patient-oriented approach, breast ultrasound, and digital mammography. In 2007 he was recognized as one of the top five breast-imaging specialists in the country.

Theodore (Ted) N. Tsangaris, MD
Medical Director of the Johns Hopkins Avon Foundation Breast Center
Chief of Breast Surgery
Associate Professor of Surgery

Dr. Tsangaris joined the Johns Hopkins faculty in March 2002 as the Medical Director of the Johns Hopkins Breast Center and Chief of Breast Surgery, Division of Surgical Oncology. He earned his BA at Wake Forest University in 1979, was awarded his MD degree at George Washington University School of Medicine in 1983, and completed his General Surgery Residency at George Washington University and his Surgical Breast Oncology Fellowship at Baylor University Medical Center in 1990. He attended Harvard School of Public Health and Harvard School of Medicine during the summer of 1994, where he completed their educational program in Clinical Effectiveness. An accomplished surgical oncologist who specializes in breast cancer, he has held several leadership positions prior to joining the Johns Hopkins faculty. These include Assistant Professor and Acting Chief of Breast Surgery at Roswell Park Cancer Institute in New York from 1990–1992; Visiting Surgical Consultant for the Saudi–U.S. University Project for King Faisal Specialist Hospital and Research Center in Saudi Arabia from 1995–1997; Director, Student Clerkships in the Department of Surgery at George Washington University Medical Center during 1995–1997, and Assistant Professor of Surgery and Director of the Breast Cancer Center at George Washington University from 1993–1997. From 1997 to February 2002, he was the Director of Breast Surgical Services and Associate Professor of Surgery at

Lombardi Cancer Center at the Georgetown University's Medical Center in Washington, DC.

Dr. Tsangaris is a nationally renowned breast surgical oncologist with expertise in surgical management as well as a breadth of knowledge and experience in clinical research in the field of breast cancer.

Kala Visvanathan, MD, MHS
Associate Professor of Epidemiology and Oncology

Dr. Visvanathan received her medical degree from the University of Sydney in Australia. She subsequently went on to complete her training in Internal Medicine and Medical Oncology at Royal Prince Alfred, a teaching hospital of the University of Sydney, and the Sidney Kimmel Comprehensive Cancer Center at Johns Hopkins. In addition, she undertook a master's in Clinical/Cancer epidemiology at the Johns Hopkins Bloomberg School of Public Health. Dr. Visvanathan currently has a joint faculty appointment in the Johns Hopkins School of Medicine and the Bloomberg School of Public Health. She is one of two physicians who run the high-risk breast and ovarian clinic at Johns Hopkins in addition to seeing cancer patients. Trained as a medical oncologist and cancer epidemiologist, Dr. Visvanathan's primary research interest is in the etiology, early detection, and prevention of breast and ovarian cancer; in particular, the evaluation of genetic, molecular, and dietary biomarkers of risk and early detection in breast cancer incidence and mortality, with an aim to modify those factors in the causal pathway with effective chemoprevention strategies.

Algorithm for Taking Care of Your Patient's Health

Emotionally

- Coping with fear of recurrence
- Differentiating between long-term side effects of therapy vs. symptoms of metasteses
- Support groups
- Stay informed about breast cancer therapy
- Psychotherapy if warranted
- Communicate with doctor about her concerns
- Participate in survivor retreats and events

Physically

- Exercise
- No smoking
- Avoid alcohol consumption
- Lymphedema prevention or management
- Nutritionally balanced diet
- Assessing risks for other types of cancers
- Stress management/yoga/relaxation

CHAPTER 1

Psycho-Oncology of Breast Cancer: Progressing into Survivorship

Lillie D. Shockney, RN, BS, MAS

What you need to know:

It is not unusual for women with breast cancer to have difficulty reengaging in their lives after their treatment has ended. This experience has been compared to the post-traumatic stress disorder experienced by some members of the military at war as well as individuals who are exposed to traumatic events.

Although most breast cancer survivors will have adjusted well after their first 2 years since diagnosis, 30% will not. These women may have issues with body image perception, fear of recurrence, sexual dysfunction, and stress disorders. In some cases you may need to refer your patient for psychotherapy to assist her with these issues.

More breast centers are offering survivor retreats for patients. These programs are designed to assist breast cancer survivors with lingering posttreatment issues.

Encouraging your patient to focus on the things she can control in her life, especially those that are health related, can greatly aid her in moving forward. These issues include weight management, smoking cessation, limiting alcohol consumption, and exercise. Encourage your patient to attend educational seminars to stay up to date on breast cancer and its treatment.

Make sure your patient is consistently getting her proper health assessments at the designated intervals, such as Pap smears, colonoscopy, physical examinations, vision checkups, blood work for monitoring her cholesterol levels, and other diagnostic assessments specific to her health issues.

Also investigate, on the patient's behalf, the availability of breast cancer support groups in her area, and refer her when you feel it is appropriate.

What your patient needs to know:

Breast cancer is a life-altering experience. It is perfectly normal to feel anxiety when treatment has ended. Fear of recurrence is particularly common for most survivors.

The patient can regain control over her life (and health) by assessing her lifestyle habits and making changes where needed to improve her overall health and reduce her risk of breast cancer recurrence.

Patients should stay informed about the latest information regarding breast cancer and its treatment. They should rely on credible sources, however, and should not believe everything they find on the Internet.

Uncertainty can result in emotional distress. The patient should be educated by you so that she can distinguish between long-term side effects of treatment and new, persistent symptoms that might signal the need for additional evaluation.

The patient should be diligent in getting her routine checkups and health evaluation tests, such as Pap smears, colonoscopy, mammograms, and physical examinations.

Patients should stay active. It is one of the best ways for anyone to keep healthy.

The patient should speak with you about any programs the breast center may offer to help her transition back into her life. Some facilities now offer survivor retreats that can prove very helpful for patients.

Support groups can be helpful as well, but only if they are effectively moderated by a trained individual who knows how to facilitate such a group.

Some women may hesitate to celebrate their survivorship for fear it will jinx them. Your patient deserves the opportunity to celebrate. If she attends breast cancer walks and other events, she will undoubtedly encounter many other survivors there.

THE PSYCHOSOCIAL TRANSITION AFTER BREAST CANCER

When a patient completes her breast cancer treatment, typically she feels more anxious than relieved (as confirmed by several studies). She is nervous about separating from her treatment team and lacks faith in her body because it has already betrayed her once. It is at this point in time her survivorship care transitions over to you. She needs to feel confident that you understand her medical and psychological needs, and can appropriately address them for her. She also does not feel confident that she is, in fact, "a survivor"; there are even debates among patients and healthcare professionals about the point at which one can refer to herself as a survivor. If the patient is still taking hormonal therapy, she is technically still being "treated"—yet we do not think of her as a patient now in active treatment.

This is a period of psychosocial transition, defined as "major life experiences that require individuals to restructure their ways of looking at the world and their plans to live in it."[1] Some studies have compared this period to the post-traumatic stress disorder experienced by some military personnel who return from combat. Helping a patient achieve posttreatment personal growth is part of the physician's responsibility in assisting the patient to move on from treatment and reengage in life in emotionally and physically healthy ways. This type of psychological growth happens when individuals making positive changes recover from a traumatic life situation.[2]

The literature documents that the majority of breast cancer survivors have adjusted well after their first 2 years since diagnosis. However, there is a subset of survivors (approximately 30%) who report psychological distress, including depression and increased anxiety, 4 years after therapy ends. In addition, a large percentage of survivors report cancer-related problems long after treatment is completed, including concerns about body image perception, fear of recurrence, post-traumatic stress disorder, and sexual dysfunction.[3] These lingering concerns can result in a woman being unable to get on with her life as a breast cancer survivor. Each ache and pain is perceived as a possible return of the cancer. This anxiety may increase as she is transitioned from seeing her oncologist to now seeing you for long-term management. Studies have confirmed that this fear of recurrence centers on the possibility of death, future treatment, and threats to health, more than issues related to roles, femininity, sexuality, or body image.[4]

During her treatment, a patient was accustomed to seeing her oncology team frequently and being reassured that she was doing well and looked fine. Initially, those visits begin to be spaced many months apart and then are discontinued completely as she transitions to your care.

COPING STRATEGIES FOR BREAST CANCER SURVIVORS

This section describes some constructive ways to help your patient regain control over her life and move on from breast cancer. The patient can assess her lifestyle habits and see if any are contributors to developing breast cancer. Smoking, alcohol consumption, weight gain, and inactivity can be considered contributors. By watching her weight, avoiding use of tobacco products (including secondary cigarette smoke), limiting alcohol consumption, and exercising regularly, your patient can feel more in control and see that she is taking charge of her health with steps that reduce the risk of breast cancer.[5,6]

Staying informed about the latest research into breast cancer and its treatment is beneficial for many breast cancer survivors. Direct your patient to Web sites that provide accurate information, and empower her so that she becomes an informed survivor. The Web site www.breastcancer.org is a useful resource, as is the Johns Hopkins site (www.hopkinsbreastcenter.org).

Some patients have difficulty returning to work and resuming their home routines, and they may need a bridge to help them for a while. There is nothing wrong with recommending that your patient consult a psychotherapist for help during this time. Breast cancer is a life-altering experience. Most marriages grow stronger when one partner has breast cancer, but some do not. Her family and coworkers may be weary after "holding down the fort" for months and, now that her treatment is done, they may expect the patient to be back to her old self and pick up all of her previous activities immediately. The patient is a different person, though—probably more in touch with her mortality. As a consequence, what she felt obligated to do before her breast cancer may seem trivial now.

Therapists and programs such as survivor retreats may help women set new life goals and figure out how to communicate with their family members about what they have experienced and how those experiences may have changed them. There is a tendency sometimes to seek a quick fix to such problems and get a prescription for antianxiety medicines. This is rarely the solution. It just numbs the patient and prevents her from dealing with the underlying cause, which needs to be discussed and dealt with openly.

Some patients experience difficulty differentiating between the long-term side effects of treatment (such as bone pain from hormonal therapy) and possible metastatic disease.

Today scans are not routinely done as part of follow-up care, but rather new-onset, persistent symptoms trigger the need for diagnostic testing (see Chapter 2). The uncertainty can result in emotional distress for women who are trying to differentiate between symptoms from previous treatment and those that represent comorbid conditions, recurrence, or normal aging. Communicating with you may help reduce the patient's uncertainty in this regard and improve her emotional and cognitive well-being.[7]

Many breast cancer survivors worry about the risk of developing other cancers, such as ovarian or colon cancer. Annual pelvic examinations, possibly periodic transvaginal ultrasounds in some cases, and colonoscopy in keeping with the standards of care recommended for other individuals will help her to feel more confident that she is doing well.

In some cases, a patient may limit her physical activity and not enjoy life as much as she could because of her fear of developing lymphedema. The advent of sentinel node biopsy has dramatically reduced this risk in the last few years. Those patients having axillary node dissections do have risks, however. One study stated that patients who have axillary node dissection could maintain their level of physical activity without an added risk of developing arm lymphedema. Having a higher body mass index (BMI) before and after the surgery appears to increase the risk of lymphedema, however.[8]

Some women experience great anxiety and guilt, fearing they may have passed this disease to their children. For women who may carry a breast cancer gene, this is a time to possibly refer them for genetic evaluation (see Chapter 6).

If your patient does carry a breast cancer gene, a genetics counselor can further assess her children's risk, if necessary. A breast cancer gene is no one's fault. This message sometimes needs to be reiterated to assuage a patient's feelings of guilt.

Anxiety about having "missed" the benefits of newer treatment options that became available after their treatment was completed is an issue for some patients. Women may read about new treatments and feel deprived because these options were not available to them. Some may attempt to find a doctor willing to give them the treatment now, even if it has been several years since their breast cancer diagnosis and treatment. Providers need to emphasize that these treatments will be available if patients need them in the future. The good news is that there are new treatments being developed on an ongoing basis that will benefit the next generation.

Encourage your patients to participate in breast cancer events that celebrate survivorship and raise money for breast cancer research. Raising money for research helps them to feel more positive about the outlook for the next generation—perhaps less treatment, and perhaps even prevention and cure.

Support groups have both good features and not-so-good features. Women who are going through active treatment can benefit from talking with others who are doing the same as well as women who have recently completed their treatment. They can feel camaraderie, a sense of belonging, and be reassured that the thoughts and fears that they are experiencing are normal. Women who attend support groups for many years, however, may not be doing themselves any favors. In one study, organized support groups were helpful to only 13% of those surveyed.[9] For some women, these groups may actually promote fear of recurrence. How effective the facilitator is in running the support group is critical to its success. If a woman is 10 years out from treatment and still feels a need to be in a support group and talk about her fears, then it may be a signal that she needs one-on-one psychotherapy.

Make your patients aware when an educational seminar is available in your area to update them on breast cancer diagnosis and treatment. Seminars keep them informed about what is the latest news regarding diagnosis, treatment, and the future as it relates to preventing and finding a cure for breast cancer.

Unfortunately, 70% of women undergoing mastectomy surgery are not offered a plastic surgery consultation to consider reconstruction. Only a small percentage of patients would not be candidates to have simultaneous reconstruction. If you are now taking care of a breast cancer survivor who had mastectomy surgery in the past without reconstruction, consider bringing up the idea up with her to see if she is interested in getting a consultation arranged. Women need permission to choose. They are so focused on the need to "get rid of the cancer" they often don't ask about reconstruction options. As more time goes by they consider it something they would not even be eligible for, when in fact they usually are. So ask her if she has thought about reconstruction and, if she opted not to do it, whether that decision was made following a consultation with a plastic surgeon. You might be surprised at the number of women that will have reconstruction done many years later by simply raising the question. Health insurance is required to cover breast reconstruction courtesy of a federal law passed in 1998. Therefore, financial barriers are no longer a rationale for not getting her silhouette whole again.

Of course, there will be women who will have chosen not to have breast reconstruction and that is fine as long as it was their personal choice. In such cases, women should be properly fitted for a breast prosthesis and mastectomy bras. Women should be refitted for breast prostheses and mastectomy bras every 2 years. Most health insurance plans help pay for 1 or 2 postsurgical garments designed for comfort and symmetry immediately following breast surgery, and 1 silicone breast prosthesis per surgical site every 24 month, and several bras each year. Refer the patient to consult her insurance provider for her specific coverage as coverage will vary. To locate a Certified Fit Specialist at an accredited facility in her area she can visit the store locator at a manufacturer's Web site, such as www.amoena.com/us.

Finally, sending your patient information via mail about self-promoting good lifestyle habits is something that patients welcome, according to a study that focused on patients' readiness to pursue lifestyle changes to improve their health.[10]

Frequently Asked Questions

1. ***What is the number one issue of concern for women after completion of their adjuvant therapy?***

   Most breast cancer survivors fear recurrence of the disease—both local recurrence and, even more so, distant recurrence that would place them in a stage IV situation. Women need a lot of reassurance regarding this issue and accurate statistics to put their risk of recurrence into perspective; otherwise, patients can end up being controlled by this disease even though they have beaten it.

2. ***What are patients' other major concerns?***

   Some patients fear that they may have passed the risk of getting breast cancer on to their children (via a breast cancer gene). Women need to be educated about genetic risk and be evaluated for it as part of their initial assessment at the time of diagnosis. The majority of women diagnosed with breast cancer will not carry the BRCA1 or BRCA2 gene; in such cases, their disease did not have a genetic origin. Helping a patient understand what the risk is for her children based on genetic risk versus not being connected to hereditary causes is important. Both the patient and her children will rest easier with this understanding. (See Chapter 6 for more information about genetic risk.)

3. ***What are constructive things women can do to reduce their risk of recurrence once they have been diagnosed and treated for breast cancer?***

   Breast cancer survivors should watch their diet—a low-fat diet is recommended. Exercise regularly. No smoking. Limit alcohol intake. Do not take hormone replacement therapy (HRT).

4. ***What are other ways to reduce anxiety about breast cancer for women who have had this disease or fear getting it?***

There is power in information. Keeping your patient informed of the latest research findings and progress related to breast cancer diagnosis, treatment, and prevention is helpful to her. Directing her to credible Web sites and newsletters about breast cancer is wise. Discourage your patient from seeking information from just any Web site, as some information found on the Internet is inaccurate and can produce more fear and misunderstanding.

REFERENCES

1. Parkes CM. Psycho-social transitions: a field for study. *Social Sci Med.* 1998;5:101–115.
2. Tedeschi RG, Calhoun LG. The Post-traumatic Growth Inventory: measuring the positive legacy of trauma. *J Traum Stress.* 1996;9:455–471.
3. Kornblith AB, Ligibel J. Psychosocial and sexual functioning of survivors of breast cancer. *Semin Oncol.* 2003;30(6):799–813.
4. Vickberg SM. The concerns about recurrence scales (CARS): a systematic measure of women's fears about the possibility of breast cancer recurrence. *Ann Behav Med.* 2003;25(1):16–24.
5. Fentiman IS, Allen DS, Hamed H. Smoking and prognosis in women with breast cancer. *Intl J Clin Pract.* 2005;59(9):999–1000.

6. Thomson CA, Flatt SW, Rock CL, et al. Increased fruit, vegetable and fiber intake and lower fat intake reported among women previously treated for invasive breast cancer. *J Am Diet Assoc.* 2002; 102(6):801–808.
7. Clayton MF, Mishel MH, Belyea M. Testing a model of symptoms, communication, uncertainty, and well-being in older breast cancer survivors. *Res Nurs Health.* 2006;29(1):18–39.
8. Johansson K, Ohlsson K, Ingvar C, et al. Factors associated with the development of arm lymphedema following breast cancer treatment: a match pair case control study. *Lymphology.* 2002;35(2);59–71.
9. Chantler M, Podbilewicz-Schuller Y, Mortimer J. Change in need for psychosocial support for women with early stage breast cancer. *J Psychosoc Oncol.* 2005; 23(2–3):65–77.
10. Demark-Wahnefried W, Peterson B, McBride C, et al. Current health behaviors and readiness to pursue life style changes among men and women diagnosed with early stage prostate and breast carcinomas. *Cancer.* 2000;88(3):674–684.

CHAPTER 2

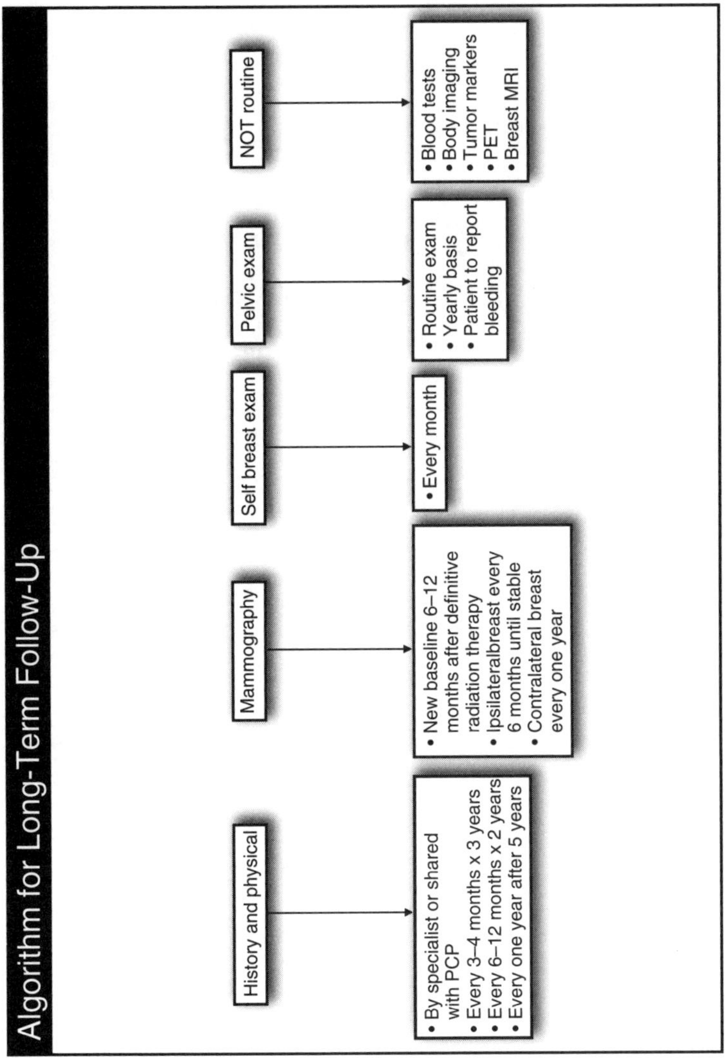
Algorithm for Long-Term Follow-Up
History and physical
• By specialist or shared with PCP
• Every 3–4 months x 3 years
• Every 6–12 months x 2 years
• Every one year after 5 years
Mammography
• New baseline 6–12 months after definitive radiation therapy
• Ipsilateralbreast every 6 months until stable
• Contralateral breast every one year
Self breast exam
• Every month
Pelvic exam
• Routine exam
• Yearly basis
• Patient to report bleeding
NOT routine
• Blood tests
• Body imaging
• Tumor markers
• PET
• Breast MRI

CHAPTER 2

Long-Term Follow-Up of Breast Cancer Survivors

Lillie D. Shockney, RN, BS, MAS
Charles Balch, MD

What you need to know:

Patients may show concern about not having scans and blood work done regularly after treatment is completed. The standard of care, however, is to rely on symptoms, and not to do scans and blood work once treatment is completed.

Patients' emotional needs may heighten during the first year after treatment is complete.

Chronic side effects may be the most worrisome issue that patients need your assistance with managing. These side effects may include peripheral neuropathy, cognitive dysfunction, and chronic joint pain.

What your patient needs to know:

The patient should make her doctor aware of any side effects she is experiencing as a result of treatment so that the physician can better address the patient's medical needs.

Although it may seem unusual, routine scans and blood tests are no longer the standard of care for monitoring patients with breast cancer and evaluating them for recurrence of their disease. Instead, the patient should report any new symptoms that linger for longer than 2 weeks. At this point, any tests will be done if they are indicated.

The time required to recover from treatment—that is, the length of time before they feel well again—varies among patients. The patient needs to give herself that time, because breast cancer is a life-altering experience. She will be working to find her "new normal" going forward.

INTRODUCTION

During the surgical and adjuvant treatment period, patients with breast cancer are seen with relative frequency by their oncology team. Most teams will see the patient every few weeks, then progress to 6-month intervals, and eventually see her annually for some period. Once a patient reaches the point that her surgery, chemotherapy, and radiation therapy are completed, she is switched to a less intensive monitoring schedule, even if she is still taking hormonal therapy. In most cases, if the patient had her wish, she would continue to see her oncology team frequently just to ensure her peace of mind, even if no tests were done. There is a sense of relief when the patient hears them say that she looks like she is doing well.

As was mentioned in the forward to this book, women with early-stage breast cancer have the same health outcomes, whether they are followed long term by you or by their oncologist.[1] Given this finding, we may see increased pressure from insurance companies to have breast cancer survivors be seen for follow-up more often by their internists or by you as a nurse practitioner and less often by their cancer specialists. Additionally, as was stated earlier in the opening of this book, the United States is facing a serious crisis—a 48% shortage of oncology specialists is anticipated to become a reality by 2020. This fact alone will force oncology doctors to transfer the follow-up care of their patients from themselves to a clinical setting with you as their survivorship care provider.

Women who survive breast cancer—and the majority will—often find themselves without an organized system for maintaining their physical and emotional health. This is an issue that many cancer organizations now recognize and that the Institute of Medicine (IOM) announced in November 2005 that it wants to address. There needs to be a definitive plan for long-term follow-up for cancer patients in general. This chapter focuses specifically on breast cancer patients and your role in functioning as one of the key healthcare providers in their long-term survivorship care.

The IOM report confirmed that there is wide variation in how physicians track and care for cancer patients once they complete their primary and adjuvant treatment. "Awareness needs to be raised for both healthcare providers and the general public. It is common now for cancer patients to finish their primary treatment unaware of their heightened health risks. They are therefore ill prepared to manage their future healthcare needs," says Dr. Sheldon Greenfield, chair of the IOM panel and director of the Center for Health Policy Research at the University of California at Irvine.[2]

The IOM report recommended that cancer patients, upon graduating from receiving care from their oncology team, have a "survivorship care plan" that provides a road map of their history of diagnosis and treatment, plus long-term follow-up recommendations for primary care providers to follow. (It also recommended that both private health insurers and Medicare/Medicaid fund such plans.) For a woman who is completing breast cancer treatment, transitioning from oncology visits to routine follow-up appointments with you, her family physician, and gynecologist is a significant milestone.

Figure 2-1 is an example of a form for recording a patient's breast cancer treatment plan. This treatment summary chart is also available on our Web site, and you are welcome to access and download the document for use in your own practice. To access a copy of this document for your personal office use, go to www.hopkinsbreastcenter.org, click on "Library," and scroll down to the document entitled "Breast Cancer Survivor Summary of Care Form."* You can download this document and save it to your computer, if you like; otherwise, you can just print blank copies as needed.

*In the "Survivorship" section, as well as the library/educational materials section, of our Web site, you will also find a document designed for patients entitled "Treatment's Done—Now What?" Feel free to review this document and provide your patients with a hard copy of it. Use the search feature as needed to explore the rest of the "Survivorship" section.

Breast Cancer Treatment Summary

Patient's name: ______________________________ **Hx #** ____________________

DOB: ____________

Date of diagnosis: ____________ **Type of breast cancer:** ________________________

Type of surgery: ____________ **Date performed:** ________________________

Pathology: ____________ **Tumor diameter (invasive component):** ___ Grade: 1 2 3

ER: _____% positive **PR:** _____% positive **Her2neu:** + ++ +++

Sentinel node status: neg pos **Total axillary nodes resected:** ____ **Total pos:** ____

Chemotherapy: Drug given ____________________ # of cycles Period of time given ________
Chemotherapy: Drug given ____________________ # of cycles Period of time given ________
Chemotherapy: Drug given ____________________ # of cycles Period of time given ________
Chemotherapy: Drug given ____________________ # of cycles Period of time given ________

Radiation: yes no **If yes:** external beam partial breast full breast chest wall axilla
Radiation: yes no **Period of time given:** ______________

Targeted therapy: Drug given ____________________ # of cycles Period of time given ________

Hormonal therapy: yes no
Drug given __________________ Start date ________ Stop date ________
Drug given __________________ Start date ________ Stop date ________
Drug given __________________ Start date ________ Stop date ________

Other drug therapies: ____
____

Recurrence: local distant **Where?** ____________________ **When?** ____________

Other pertinent information: ____
____
____
____
____

Name of breast surgeon: ________________________ **Contact #:** ______________
Address: ________________________
____

Name of medical oncologist: ________________________ **Contact #:** ______________
Address: ________________________
____

Name of radiation oncologist: ________________________ **Contact #:** ______________
Address: ________________________
____

FIGURE 2-1

It is recommended that you obtain copies of the patient's medical records directly from her oncology team, rather than relying solely on the patient being the source of this important medical information. Although some patients are excellent historians and provide accurate information about their treatment history, others (as you undoubtedly know) are not.

The breast cancer treatment plan summary is a document that can "grow" with the patient, particularly if you are also seeing her during her active treatment. If you are assuming her posttreatment care, then this tool serves as the starting point for understanding her breast cancer history, prognostic information, and treatment she has completed. Figure 2-2 shows a breast cancer treatment plan summary for one patient.

LONG-TERM NEEDS OF PATIENTS WITH BREAST CANCER

Your patient's biggest worry is recurrence of her breast cancer. The majority of women who are diagnosed and treated for breast cancer live a normal life span. Although the incidence of breast cancer has risen from year to year in the last 15 to 20 years, the mortality rate has decreased. Women who have had breast cancer are at risk of getting the disease again and usually are aware of this fact. Twenty-five percent of women previously diagnosed with breast cancer will face the prospect of hearing "You have breast cancer again."

It is important to note that women who do get breast cancer again in the ipsilateral breast or contralateral breast do *not* have a worse prognosis or higher mortality than those who

Breast Cancer Treatment Summary

Patient's name: Jane Doe **Hx #** 12345 **DOB:** 10/20/1964

Date of diagnosis: 2/10/2009 **Type of breast cancer:** Invasive ductal + DCIS

Type of surgery: Lumpectomy with sentinel node biopsy **Date performed:** 2/21/2009

Pathology: 1.8 cm total **Tumor diameter (invasive component):** 1.3 cm Grade: 1 2 (3)

ER: 90 % positive **PR:** 80 % positive **Her2neu:** (+) ++ +++

Sentinel node status: (neg) pos **Total axillary nodes resected:** 1 **Total pos:** 0

Chemotherapy: Drug given Adriamycin 4 # of cycles Period of time given 3/09 – 5/09
Chemotherapy: Drug given ____ # of cycles Period of time given ____
Chemotherapy: Drug given ____ # of cycles Period of time given ____
Chemotherapy: Drug given ____ # of cycles Period of time given ____

Radiation: (yes) no **If yes:** (external beam) partial breast (full breast) chest wall axilla
Radiation: yes no **Period of time given:** 6/09 – 7/09

Targeted therapy: Drug given none # of cycles Period of time given ____

Hormonal therapy: (yes) no
Drug given Tamoxifen Start date 8/09 Stop date ____
Drug given ____ Start date ____ Stop date ____
Drug given ____ Start date ____ Stop date ____

Other drug therapies: ____

Recurrence: local distant **Where?** ____ **When?** ____

Other pertinent information: ____

Name of breast surgeon: Dr. Thomas Operation **Contact #:** (444) 555-1100
Address: 11 Surgical Road
Anywhere, USA

Name of medical oncologist: Dr. Mary Medicine **Contact #:** (444) 555-2200
Address: 14 Chemo Street
Anywhere, USA

Name of radiation oncologist: Dr. Stephen Zap **Contact #:** (444) 555-3333
Address: Exray Parkway
Anywhere, USA

FIGURE 2-2

do not develop local recurrence or a new primary tumor. The younger she is, however, the longer her life and thus the greater her potential to be among the 25% of patients who reexperience this disease. Statistically, there is a 0.5% to 1.0% risk per year of a new contralateral breast cancer in these patients. Ipsilateral breast cancer recurrence may have the same prognosis as a new primary tumor in patients who previously had breast-conserving surgery.

Another potential risk is the development of swelling (lymphedema) of the arm or breast. This problem occurs in 5% to 20% of women, with the risk depending on the degree to which the lymph channel draining the arm or the breast was interrupted after more extensive (radical) removal of the lymph glands in the armpit; the risk is greater if there was also radiation therapy to the armpit. For more information, see the American Society of Clinical Oncology (ASCO) Web site for patients (www.plwc.org) or the National Lymphedema Network Web site (www.lymphnet.org).

TAKING CARE OF THE WHOLE PATIENT

Taking care of breast cancer survivors involves more than just providing breast health follow-up. Rather, it means addressing the needs of the whole patient—both physical and emotional.

The leading cause of death in women older than 50 years of age remains heart disease. Although a breast cancer survivor may not be concerned about heart disease, she should be—if only because having had breast cancer does not make her immune to cardiovascular conditions. In some cases, her risk may actually have increased because of the side effects of some drugs used for treatment of her breast cancer. While a woman is going through her breast cancer treatment, sometimes there are lapses or delays in her annual or semiannual general health assessment. Assessments so affected may include her annual physical examination and gynecological examination; even eye examinations can fall off the radar screen.

The breast cancer survivor also has an increased risk of developing other types of cancers. In particular, the risk of ovarian cancer is higher for women with a diagnosis of breast cancer. Patients with breast cancer may also be at increased risk of developing other types of cancers such as colon cancer (see Chapter 6). Women who are taking tamoxifen should have annual pelvic examinations and Pap smears. If they report abnormal vaginal bleeding or spotting or other pelvic symptoms that cannot be explained, they may need further evaluation with transvaginal ultrasound or endometrial biopsy to rule out uterine cancer, as this condition is a known complication for a small percentage of women taking this hormonal therapy.

In addition, women on tamoxifen have a risk of blood clots. Thus a patient reporting unilateral leg pain, chest pain, shortness of breath, or other symptoms should be evaluated for deep vein thrombosis or blood clots. In some cases, liver function tests may change while taking this hormonal therapy as well. Patients also need symptom management for hot flashes and possible depression (see Chapter 5).

Premenopausal women who have had ovarian failure associated with adjuvant therapy (chemotherapy) and postmenopausal women who are being treated with aromatase inhibitors (AIs) are at increased risk of developing osteopenia or osteoporosis; these conditions are associated with an increased risk of bone fracture. Bone health monitoring and bone loss prevention, therefore, need to be included in the patient's long-term management. If hormonal therapy with an AI is considered in women who have experienced amenorrhea following treatment, baseline levels of estradiol and gonadotropin should be obtained before the AI therapy begins, and the nurse practitioner should subsequently perform serial monitoring of these hormone levels. For women who had bilateral oophorectomies before starting AI therapy, these blood tests are not necessary.

It is also important to assess your patient for adherence to long-term hormonal therapy, as compliance has proven to be an issue for breast cancer patients. Because the side effects associated with such therapy may overwhelm these patients, they may decide to skip or alter their dosing schedules in an effort to obtain symptom relief. This is a time to help them with reducing these side effects as well as to reiterate the purpose of the endocrine therapy. The goal is to keep these patients on track over the long term with the intended treatment regimen.

Many patients with breast cancer report feeling depressed after treatment is completed. In some cases, the depression may be related to losing the oncology team the patient saw as her touchstone, or it may be caused by side effects of hormone suppression, body image changes, or other feelings of loss (e.g., hair loss, symptoms of sexual dysfunction). Inquiring about the patient's emotional health needs to be part of every routine examination; you should not leave it up to the patient to bring up these concerns.

As described in the ASCO Web site for patients (Healthy Living After Cancer; www.plwc.org), women recovering from breast cancer are encouraged to follow established guidelines for good health. After a cancer diagnosis, many survivors may want to make changes such as eating better, exercising more, and finding better ways to manage stress. Although practicing healthy habits is important for everyone, it is especially important for cancer survivors because they can be at an increased risk for other health problems—for example, obesity, heart problems, diabetes, or bone weakness (osteoporosis)—as a result of their cancer treatment.

Patients need to talk with you to develop a plan that is best for their needs. Moderate physical activity can help them rebuild their strength and energy levels. Nurses should be prepared to help their patients create a safe exercise plan based upon each patient's unique needs, physical abilities, and fitness level.

ASSESSING PATIENTS FOR DISTANT RECURRENCE

Monitoring practices for metastatic disease vary widely among oncology specialists. There is general agreement on the need for physical examination every 3 to 6 months during the first 5 years and annual examinations thereafter. However, there are mixed views regarding which routine tests are beneficial. Some providers order complete blood counts (CBCs), blood chemistries, and even blood tumor markers such as CA 27.29, carcinoembryonic antigen (CEA), and CA 15-3. The problem with the blood markers is that they are not sufficiently sensitive or specific to warrant their routine use in all patients. The most common marker used for breast cancer patients has been CA 27.29, which measures the presence of an abnormal protein associated with some cancer cell production.

Women who have had lumpectomy surgery and/or who have a remaining healthy breast should continue to receive mammograms. A new baseline mammogram is needed on the treated breast within 4 to 8 weeks after radiation is completed. Posttherapy follow-up is optimally performed initially by members of the patient's treatment team and should include regular physical examinations and mammograms. For women who are undergoing breast-conserving therapy, the first follow-up mammogram should be performed approximately 6 months after the completion of her radiation therapy.

National Comprehensive Cancer Network (NCCN) guidelines do not support routine ultrasound to screen the breast in asymptomatic patients. The use of dedicated breast magnetic resonance imaging (MRI) may be considered for posttherapy surveillance and follow-up in women who are considered to be at high risk of bilateral disease, such as BRCA gene carriers; the incidence of bilateral breast cancer is higher in women who carry the BRCA1 or BRCA2 gene. There is no evidence of any benefit from performing other imaging studies, such as bone scans, computerized axial tomography (CAT) scans, chest x-rays, or positron emission tomography (PET) scans, on a routine monitoring basis.

Bone density tests should be performed in women who are taking an AI or having some form of ovarian suppression or ablation. Be sure that your patient understands that a bone density test is not a bone scan and is not being done to look for metastatic disease.

A point of frustration for patients is the issue of not doing scans and tests on a routine scheduled basis. Some women prefer to have x-rays of some type periodically, even though they have anxiety about hearing the results. Based on information gathered by ASCO and the NCCN, there does not appear to be a survival benefit to finding the disease on a scan before a patient reports new symptoms of possible metastatic disease. Conversely, the ability to control the disease within the breast is surely improved, regardless of survival outcome. Studies published as early as 1994 confirmed that there was no impact on survival by doing intensive monitoring versus routine monitoring of patients.[3] Despite these findings, some providers still opt to perform scans and measure blood tumor markers, although these measures are usually reserved for their patients who are at high risk for relapse or second breast cancer (e.g., those with locally advanced disease) and are employed less often for women who have early-stage breast cancers.

Do not be surprised if at the time of the patient transitioning to you she requests scans during your first consultation with her. It is a sign of her anxiety level and need for reassurance that she will be appropriately monitored and cared for by you.

PATIENTS REPORTING CHRONIC FATIGUE AND REDUCTION IN PHYSICAL ACTIVITY

As many as one third of women treated for breast cancer have reported symptoms of fatigue lasting as long as 10 years after their diagnosis. The incidence was higher in women with cardiovascular problems and depressive symptoms and in those who were treated with combined radiation and chemotherapy. Although it is recognized as a subjective symptom, fatigue can be so debilitating that it affects the patient's quality of life and performance of activities of daily living.

In one study, researchers found that, much like in the first 5-year interval after diagnosis, 34% of women reported fatigue symptoms 5 to 10 years after their initial diagnosis.[4] Approximately 21% complained of fatigue at both time intervals.

Another study demonstrated that women who survived breast cancer accounted for nearly half of all female cancer survivors.[5] Overall these women reported high levels of health, physical functioning, and emotional well-being. Their energy level and social functioning remained the same as they were at the 5-year post-diagnosis mark and the 9.5-year remeasurement phase. In the follow-up study period, women reported less frequent hot flashes, night sweats, vaginal discharge, and breast sensitivity than they had experienced before. When the authors of this study looked at the late effects of chemotherapy, tamoxifen, or a combination of both therapies on quality of life, they found a statistically significant decrease in physical functioning associated with adjuvant therapy, even many years after the treatment ended.[5]

RECOMMENDED TESTS FOR LONG-TERM FOLLOW-UP CARE

The following tests are recommended for survivors of breast cancer:

- Annual mammography (for women who have not had bilateral mastectomies)

- Other routine cancer screening as appropriate for age and risk factors—colon, cervix, uterus
- Regular clinic visits for history and physical examination:
    - Years 1–3: every 3 to 4 months
    - Years 3–5: every 6 months
    - Subsequent follow-up annually
- Healthcare maintenance: bone and cardiovascular health
- No routine tests—rely on new development of symptoms to trigger tests to be done
- Clinical breast examination annually by a gynecologist or primary care provider (PCP)

The following tests are not currently recommended by ASCO for regular follow-up care because they have not been shown to lengthen the life of a person with breast cancer:

- CBC and liver and kidney function tests
- Chest x-ray
- Bone scan
- Liver ultrasound
- CT or CAT scan
- Fluorodeoxyglucose-positron emission tomography (FDG-PET) scan
- Breast MRI
- Breast cancer blood tumor markers, such as CA 15-3, CA 27.29, and CEA

Frequently Asked Questions

1. ***What were the findings from the ASCO Expert Panel regarding surveillance of breast cancer patients?***

   The evidence supported the contention that the cornerstone for appropriate breast cancer follow-up is a regular history, physical examination, and mammography. The patient's history and physical examination should be performed by a physician who is experienced in the surveillance of cancer patients. Examination frequency should be as follows: every 3 to 6 months for the first 3 years, every 6 to 12 months for years 4 and 5, and then annually thereafter. Patients who are at high risk for familial breast cancer should be referred to a genetic counselor for risk assessment. For women who have had breast-conserving surgery, a posttreatment mammogram should be performed 1 year after the initial mammogram and at least 6 months after completion of radiation therapy. Routine tests are not recommended in asymptomatic patients.[6]

2. ***My patient prefers to have a breast MRI rather than an annual mammogram because her breast cancer originally was not seen on a mammogram. Is this acceptable?***

   No, the standard of practice for breast cancer detection remains mammography. If the radiologist following her breast imaging studies believes that an MRI would be beneficial as an additional study to rule out or more clearly define something seen or felt, then MRI is used. MRI is not intended as a substitute for mammography, including for women with dense breast tissue.

3. ***My patient has requested that she have blood drawn to evaluate for tumor markers at least every 6 months. She tells me it will reduce her anxiety if she can see that her blood results are remaining in the normal range.***

   Tumor marker evaluation is not part of the standard guidelines for long-term follow-up and may be elevated for reasons unrelated to cancer recurrence. Because of their imperfect sensitivity and specificity, tumor markers are *not* routinely used to monitor patients for cancer recurrence. Educating your patient about this may help reduce her desire to have these tests. The downside of such tests is that the results may come back elevated without a known cause, which can increase her anxiety without good reason.

4. ***My patient was on Herceptin. Do I need to perform routine cardiac tests on her over the long term?***

   No, such tests are performed only if the patient develops new symptoms that trigger a need to evaluate her cardiac status. The oncologist should have performed left ventricular ejection fraction evaluations during her treatment and upon completion of her therapy.

5. ***I do not know my patient's treatment plan for her breast cancer, and I do not feel that she is a good historian for this information. How important is it to know these details?***

   Pretty important. You always want to know your patient's medical history, and this treatment is a very significant component. It is important for you to include in her medical record information about chemotherapy drugs that may have affected the patient's heart and the results of her last cardiac tests. Even knowing the details of the stage of her disease and, therefore, her risk of recurrence is necessary for you to provide your patient with appropriate care. If you do not have this information, contact her breast surgeon, medical oncologist, and radiation oncologist. Ideally in the coming years, as the IOM has recommended, a specific summary of this information will be provided to both the patient and to you as her long-term cancer survivor doctor.

6. ***Where can I find more information and stay updated on changes related to the guidelines for long-term follow-up of breast cancer patients?***

   Go to www.asco.org or www.nccn.org for the latest information on this subject. The ASCO Web site, www.plwc.org, is a good source for patients.

REFERENCES

1. Grunfeld E, Levine MN, Julian JA, et al. Randomized trial of long-term follow-up for early stage breast cancer: a comparison of family physicians versus specialists care. *J Clin Oncol.* 2006;24(6):848–855.
2. Institute of Medicine. *From cancer patient to cancer survivor: lost in transition.* Washington, DC: The National Academies Press; 2005.
3. Roselli Del Turco M, Palli D, Cariddi A, et al. The efficacy of intense follow-up testing in breast cancer cases. *Ann Oncol.* 1995;6(suppl 2):37–39.
4. Rodgers A. Routine follow-up of breast cancer in primary care. *BMJ.* 1997;314:1129–1130.
5. Ganz PA, Desmond KA, Leedham B, et al. Quality of life in long-term disease-free survivors of breast cancer: a follow-up study. *J Natl Cancer Inst.* 2002;94:39–49.
6. Khatcheressian JL, Wolff A, Smith T, et al., for the ASCO Breast Cancer Surveillance Expert Panel. 2006 Update of Breast Cancer Follow-Up and Management Guideline in Adjuvant Setting. *J Clin Oncol.* 2006;24:5091–5097.

CHAPTER 3

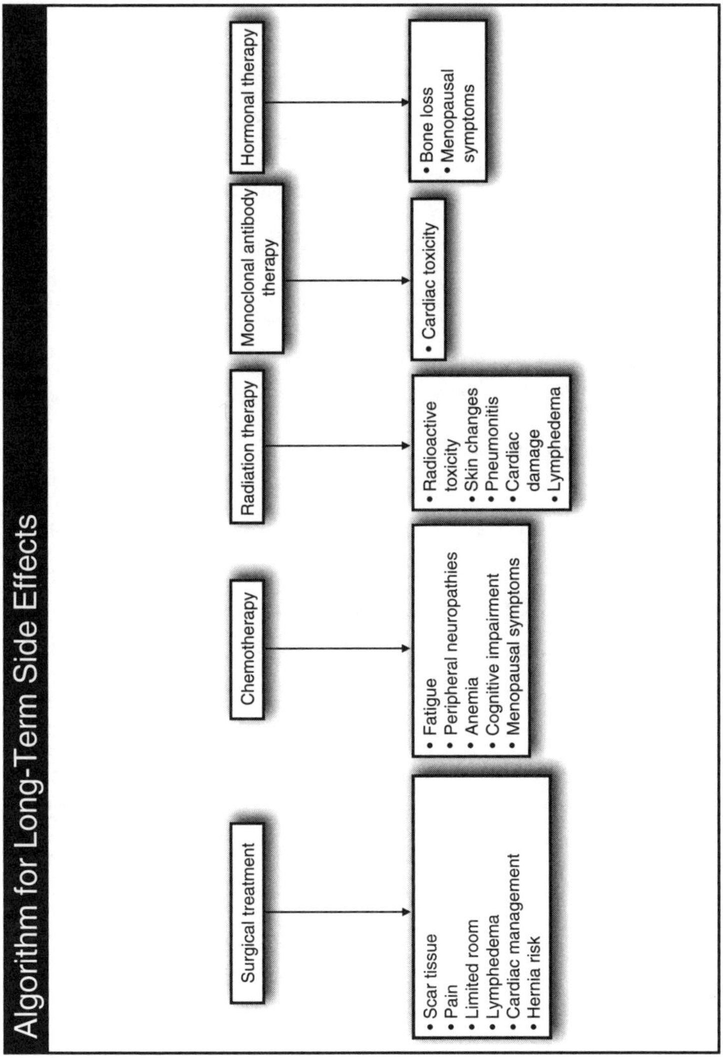
Algorithm for Long-Term Side Effects
Surgical treatment
• Scar tissue
• Pain
• Limited room
• Lymphedema
• Cardiac management
• Hernia risk
Chemotherapy
• Fatigue
• Peripheral neuropathies
• Anemia
• Cognitive impairment
• Menopausal symptoms
Radiation therapy
• Radioactive toxicity
• Skin changes
• Pneumonitis
• Cardiac damage
• Lymphedema
Monoclonal antibody therapy
• Cardiac toxicity
Hormonal therapy
• Bone loss
• Menopausal symptoms

CHAPTER 3

Management of Long-Term Side Effects

Lillie D. Shockney, RN, BS, MAS

What you need to know:

Patients can be frustrated with the continuation or even new onset of side effects that occur as a result of the treatment they have completed in the past (radiation) or may still be receiving long term (hormonal therapy). Control of side effects can only be attempted if the patient is open with you in telling you her symptoms. Working with your patient to help her have a good quality of life while continuing to experience and work on reducing side effects from treatment is one of the goals. Premenopausal women have potentially a longer period of life ahead of them to deal with long-term side effects, specially those associated with menopausal management. Providing your patient an opportunity to discuss her lingering side effects as well as to be assessed for the potential development of new symptoms should take place with each physical examination.

What your patient needs to know:

Side effects from some treatments can continue for an extended period of time after treatment has been completed. Making you aware of these symptoms is the patient's responsibility. It is important that she inform you of these side effects and not attempt to seek a remedy for them independent of medical judgment. Advice for management of these symptoms and control of them should be prescribed only by the healthcare professionals involved in her long-term management and care.

SURGICAL TREATMENT

SCAR TISSUE

Some patients can experience tightening of their scars over time. This can be due to effects of radiation, lack of exercising to stretch out incisions after surgical treatment, the body's tendencies to form keloids, or even from gaining weight. There are some situations that this is painful or limiting the range of motion to the degree that surgical revisions are needed. Referring the patient to a breast plastic surgeon may be considered.

PAIN

Following mastectomy without reconstruction or lumpectomy with radiation, some women experience chronic pain, sensory discomfort, or phantom limb sensation. In some cases it may require treatment to control with analgesics, nerve blocks, or other methods.

LIMITED RANGE OF MOTION

This can be especially problematic for patients who have undergone axillary node dissections and did not regain their range of motion and arm strength after their surgery was completed. Though by the time that you are now seeing her as a survivor who has completed treatment, if you note this problem, consider referring the patient to rehab medicine for evaluation and treatment.

LYMPHEDEMA

For patients who have undergone axillary node dissection and/or have had radiation to their axillae, risk of lymphedema can be a chronic concern. The risk of developing lymphedema does not diminish with time. The patient will always be at risk of developing this chronic condition. Needle sticks (due to puncturing the skin) and blood pressure measurements (due to constriction) should be avoided. If swelling of the arm is noted, referral to a rehab medicine expert therapist in lymphedema management and prevention is warranted.

MICROVASCULAR FLAP RECONSTRUCTIONS AND LINK TO CARDIAC MANAGEMENT

The presence or risk of developing cardiovascular disease in the future due to family history or personal risk factors can influence the plastic surgeon's selection of vessels when DIEP flap or S-GAP reconstruction was performed. This is also noteworthy for patients you may be caring for who are considering having delayed flap reconstruction several or even many years after their original mastectomy surgery was performed. The recipient vessels where free flaps are transferred were traditionally the thoracodorsal artery and vein in the axilla. These vessels were often dissected and preserved during axillary dissections and easily accessible from the mastectomy defect. Increasingly, the choice of recipient vessels is the internal mammary (IM) artery and vein. The IM artery is the same vessel that cardiac surgeons use for coronary revascularization for patients with cardiovascular disease. You as well as your patient needs to inform her cardiologist and cardiothoracic surgeon if in the future she needs a coronary artery bypass graft (CABG) procedure.

HERNIA RISK

This is a potential problem for women who have had TRAM flap reconstruction. The abdominal muscles were severed in order to tunnel up the abdomen fat to recreate the breast. This causes the abdomen to be prone to hernia and to bulge whenever something heavy is lifted. Usually patients are discouraged from lifting more than 20 pounds for the rest of their lives. This can be very difficult, however, from the perspective of daily living, so risk is clearly there. She should be assessed for bulging or hernia symptoms each time she is seen by you. If hernia does occur, commonly it is the plastic surgeon who performed the TRAM flap that surgically repairs this.

CHEMOTHERAPY

FATIGUE

Fatigue is common during breast cancer treatment and one of the most debilitating side effects. The severity may vary, but most women do experience fatigue at some point during or after treatment. The exact cause of fatigue during chemotherapy is not clearly known. Some patients continue to experience fatigue after their treatment has been completed, even months or years later. Assessment of the patient for the cause of the continued fatigue is important. Evaluating her for anemia and clinical depression are two particular issues to assess.

There has been a wealth of research on fatigue that supports the use of moderate exercise or physical activity during chemotherapy. A brisk walk for 15 to 30 minutes, 5 days a week, has been shown to improve physical fitness and allows patients to perform activities of daily living.[1,2] It is important for healthcare providers to explain the benefits of exercise and to encourage patients to increase physical activity to improve their overall health and well-being. A patient may have been inactive for an extended period of time, depending on the types of treatments she received. Helping her to be motivated to improve her physical activity is an important role for you to fulfill.

PERIPHERAL NEUROPATHIES

Certain chemotherapy medications can cause peripheral neuropathies. In general, this side effect is temporary and most patients return to normal once the treatment is completed. In some patients this side effect can be permanent, however, which is why it is being brought to your attention. So, careful evaluation and monitoring is important. If peripheral neuropathy does become a problem, treatment with medications, such as Neurontin, may help reduce the associated discomfort. The patient may already be on this medication when she is transitioned to you.

ANEMIA

Anemia is a rare complication of adjuvant treatment for breast cancer, but it is seen more commonly in patients being treated chronically for metastatic disease. In some cases, anemia may continue to be a problem after treatment is completed. Lack of iron, vitamin B_{12}, and folic acid may also cause anemia, so check the patient's levels periodically.

COGNITIVE IMPAIRMENT (CHEMO BRAIN)

It is estimated that 18% to 82% of cancer patients who receive standard-dose chemotherapy will develop some cognitive impairment. This includes memory loss, inability to concentrate, inability to perform multiple tasks, and others. Although most of these symptoms improve in just a few months after treatment, cognitive impairment has been observed for 2 years or longer after treatment was completed.

The exact cause is likely multifactorial—that is, chemotherapy, hormonal therapy, stress, depression, and menopause. Although patients have been complaining of this side effect for years, little is known about its exact cause, prevalence, or treatment. Cognitive impairment has only recently begun being investigated. There are multiple ongoing trials that will answer some of these questions. For those patients with cognition impairment that lingers after treatment is completed, reassessing their cognitive functioning when you are performing an annual physical examination is important. Memory problems are frustrating for patients; however, it is somewhat reassuring that most symptoms will completely resolve shortly after treatment is completed.

MENOPAUSE OR MENOPAUSAL SYMPTOMS

Of all the side effects that a patient might experience as a result of her breast cancer treatment, menopausal symptoms are usually the most frustrating to the patient. They can directly impact her quality of life for an extended period of time. For some patients, this can be an ongoing issue for years.

Chemotherapy in premenopausal women can often cause women to enter menopause temporarily while receiving treatment or permanently, long after treatment is done. These women can experience premature menopausal symptoms, which can be psychologically and physically difficult. Evidence suggests that treatment with estrogen may increase the risk of breast cancer recurrence, so management of these symptoms becomes a challenge.[3] Many women have severe and sometimes debilitating hot flashes. There is evidence that selective serotonin reuptake inhibitors (SSRIs) such as venlafaxine, paroxetine, or fluoxetine may decrease the intensity of hot flashes by 45% to 60%.[4] There have been few studies of herbal treatments with breast cancer patients. Randomized trials with soy products failed to demonstrate a significant improvement in hot flash symptoms when compared to placebo. Similar results were reported from a study randomizing breast cancer patients to black cohosh or placebo. The safety of these products has not been demonstrated for use in the breast cancer population, as the phytoestrogens may stimulate breast cancer and antagonize the antitumor effects of tamoxifen.[5] Vaginal dryness is another common menopausal symptom that is difficult to manage. In some cases, it can be successfully treated with over-the-counter vaginal lubricants. In other patients, however, this does not relieve the symptoms, and the use of local or topical estrogen therapy is very effective. However, some estrogen is systemically absorbed with this route, and there are no data to assess the safety of topical estrogen use in patients with breast cancer. Although the exact risk is not known, some women are willing to take on this risk to improve their quality of life.

CARDIOMYOPATHY

For patients who have received Adriamycin, a small number will develop cardiac toxicity as a complication. MUGA scans or echocardiograms would have been performed at specific intervals while receiving this chemotherapy drug. If cardiomyopathy was diagnosed, then she will continue to need to be followed by a cardiologist as well as being seen by you. Work closely with her cardiologist to avoid duplication of tests and procedures. Out of anxiety, patients sometimes may ask multiple healthcare providers to order various tests for them. Coordination of care is important here. If she reports an increase in shortness of breath, difficulty climbing stairs that is new, chest pain, or other symptoms, these new findings should be promptly assessed.

RADIATION TREATMENT

RADIATION TOXICITY

Radiation therapy, although beneficial in improving both local control and survival, is not without physical costs. The physical costs may include rib, lung, nerve, and soft-tissue damage. It is important to note that toxic effects of radiation can be affected by several treatment and patient-related factors. Treatment-related factors include type and energy of radiation, area treated, dose, fraction size, immobilization devices, and dosimetric plans.[6,7] Patient-related factors associated with increased toxicity include body mass index (BMI), concurrent chemotherapy, comorbidities (e.g., diabetes, connective tissue diseases, renal failure, smoking), and previous radiation exposure. Side effects or toxicities can be separated into two general categories: early and late. Early (or acute) toxicities occur during the course of radiation; late toxicities may occur 6 weeks to several years after radiation. The most common acute side effects from whole-breast radiation are fatigue and skin irritation. The severity and incidence of these side effects and all others vary greatly from patient to patient, however. The fatigue tends to be very mild such that many women are able to continue working full-time during the course of treatment. Skin irritation, or radiation dermatitis, is also fairly common. In some studies, as many as 90% of patients have developed some form of radiation dermatitis.

SKIN CHANGES: SHRINKAGE, FIRMNESS, PIGMENTATION

Late breast-related side effects associated with whole-breast radiation may include breast shrinkage, fibrosis, edema, telangiectasias, hypopigmentation/hyperpigmentation, and tenderness.[7,8] The deep layer of the epidermis contains basal stem cells. These stem cells are responsible for maintaining the cells that make up the cornified layer of the epidermis. Radiation damages these stem cells. As a consequence, there is shedding of the cornified layer (dry desquamation). The radiation therapy may also cause capillary dilatation, increased permeability, and an inflammatory response resulting in erythema and edema. There is also hyperpigmentation from migration of the melanocytes to the surface. Radiation-induced epilation, plus loss of sweat and sebaceous glands, results in dry and pruritic skin. With continued loss of the basal cell layer, the dermis will then be exposed (moist desquamation), which may progress to frank ulceration.

Healing entails reepithelialization via repopulation of the residual basal cells or migration of basal cells from neighboring areas.[8,9] Late effects of this skin damage may include decreased skin integrity, telangiectasias, and change in pigmentation.

A multitude of putative treatments are available. Unfortunately, very few have been proven to be more effective than the best supportive care in clinical trials. Putative therapies include washing with mild soap, use of aloe, barrier films, corticosteroids, antimicrobial creams (silver sulfadiazide), and trolamine. Two of these treatments have been studied in a prospective fashion and found to be somewhat effective. In a randomized prospective trial, *Calendula officinalis* cream was found to significantly reduce skin toxicity when compared to trolamine.[9] Trolamine has been shown to be no better than the best supportive care. Hyaluronic acid cream, when compared in a randomized prospective trial to placebo, was found to significantly delay the onset of severe skin toxicity.[10] Although ensuring a reduction in skin toxicity is a laudable goal, given the lack of effective agents one should at minimum provide supportive care including, if possible, pain relief.

PNEUMONITIS

Due to their proximity to the treated breast, other organs and structures may also be affected by radiation-induced toxicities. One such toxicity is radiation pneumonitis, which is characterized by interstitial inflammation associated with a nonproductive cough and/or low-grade fever.

The risk of developing radiation pneumonitis ranges from 1% to 7% and has been linked to patient- and treatment-related factors such as obesity and radiation dose and fields.[11–15] Chemotherapy may also increase the risk of developing radiation pneumonitis. A short course of corticosteroids followed by a slow taper has been used successfully at our institution to treat this condition.

CARDIAC DAMAGE

With left breast/chest wall treatment, there is a risk of radiation exposure to the heart. Meta-analyses of studies using outdated radiation techniques have shown an increased rate of cardiac events in participants who received radiation compared to those who did not.[16] This increase in cardiac events did not become obvious until 15 years after therapy. With modern radiation machines and techniques, however, there is little evidence to suggest increased cardiac morbidity with radiation. For example, in the three modern PMXRT trials in which the chest wall and supraclavicular (SCV), axillary, and internal mammary lymph nodes were treated, there was no statistically significant difference in cardiac morbidity.[7,11,17] As the use of systemic chemotherapy increases, especially with agents known to be cardiotoxic (e.g., anthracyclines and trastuzamab), it is necessary to remain vigilant in avoiding and assessing the potential for radiation-induced cardiac toxicity.

LYMPHEDEMA

Lymphedema is perhaps one of the most feared late effects of radiation therapy. The definition of lymphedema varies greatly in the literature, which inherently makes comparisons between studies and reporting the true incidence extremely difficult. At our institution, we define lymphedema as a greater than 2-cm circumference difference between the affected and nonaffected arm measured at 10 cm above and below the olecranon. This is not a universally accepted definition. Some define lymphedema as a cumulative difference of more than 10 cm between these measurements, whereas others look for a difference in volume measured by water displacement when the arm is placed in a water bath.

In part as a consequence of the failure to reach a universally accepted definition of lymphedema, reported rates of this condition vary greatly. The highest rates appear to be associated with a full axillary dissection (levels I–III) combined with axillary radiation therapy.[18] Other factors associated with an increased risk of lymphedema include obesity, age, hypertension, infection, radiation fields and dose, number of nodes removed, and number of nodes containing metastatic disease.[19–23] Fortunately, rates appear to have dropped significantly with the advent of sentinel node biopsies, limited nodal dissection (levels I–II only), and judicious use of modern radiation techniques. In the PMXRT randomized trials, lymphedema was seen in only 9–14% of the patients.[17]

The modern incidence of lymphedema is probably in the range of 10% to 20%.

There is no cure for lymphedema. Instead, intervention is motivated by the desire to palliate symptoms and reduce risk of complications. Management of lymphedema includes massage, sequential compression, and compressive garments.[24] In addition, patients are instructed to avoid infections, blood draws, and blood pressure screening in the at-risk arm. We recommend that the patient be seen by a lymphedema specialist at the earliest sign of lymphedema.

SECONDARY MALIGNANCIES

Another feared and often-mentioned potential side effect of radiation is the development of a second, nonbreast malignancy. Approximately 7% to 8% of women undergoing adjuvant radiation for breast cancer will develop a second malignancy; nevertheless, when compared to similar patients who did not undergo radiation treatment, there does not appear to be a statistically significant difference in the development of a secondary malignancy or, if one exists, it is quite small. [25,26] Although Obedian et al.[25] and Woodward et al.[26] found no overall statistically significant difference, Galper et al.[27] reported a 1% absolute increase in second, nonbreast malignancies associated with radiation therapy. Of note, however, is the apparent increase in lung cancer in women who smoke and receive radiation therapy. Galper et al. reported a 15-year risk of developing lung cancer of 0.3%, 4.7%, and 6% in women who never smoked, who stopped smoking at diagnosis of breast cancer, and who continued to smoke after completing radiation, respectively.

Other late side effects of radiation therapy with standard fractionation include brachial plexopathy (1%), spontaneous rib weakening or fracture (2% to 3%), decreased shoulder mobility (5%), and grade 2 breast fibrosis (4%).[12,13]

MONOCLONAL ANTIBODY THERAPY

The most serious side effect associated with trastuzumab, one of the monoclonal antibodies, is cardiac dysfunction, defined as overt congestive heart failure (CHF), cardiomyopathy, or a 10% or greater decrease in the left ventricular ejection fraction (LVEF). This problem occurs in approximately 5% of patients who are treated with trastuzumab monotherapy, in approximately 14% of patients who receive trastuzumab in combination with paclitaxel, and in more than 25% of patients who receive trastuzumab concurrently with an anthracycline (the baseline rate with anthracycline therapy is about 8%). This high rate of cardiac toxicity with concomitant anthracycline and trastuzumab therapy led the FDA to approve trastuzumab in combination with paclitaxel, but not anthracyclines.

Additional risk factors for trastuzumab-related cardiac toxicity include age older than 60 years, prior anthracycline therapy such that the cumulative dose exceeds 400 mg/m^2, preexisting cardiac disease, and prior chest wall radiation therapy.

The cardiac toxicity associated with trastuzumab is typically reversible. This characteristic distinguishes this side effect from the known cardiac toxicity associated with anthracycline therapy, which is typically irreversible. Anthracycline cardiac toxicity is associated with clear structural damage to the heart muscle, with myofibrillar disarray being seen on endomyocardial biopsy. In contrast, in patients who are treated with trastuzumab, the myocardium appears normal. The vast majority of patients who develop cardiac dysfunction while on trastuzumab have symptoms and signs of CHF, and improve with standard therapy for CHF. Most oncologists hold trastuzumab at the onset of cardiac dysfunction, and then cautiously reintroduce the drug once the patient has improved after taking heart failure therapy.

HORMONAL THERAPY

Your patient may still be on hormonal therapy when she transitions to you for long-term survivorship care. Chapter 5 covers hormonal therapy and provides you more information about this specific adjuvant treatment that is recommended for survivors with hormone receptor-positive tumors. Treatment can range from 5 to 10 years. If your patient is on hormonal therapy, please read Chapter 5 carefully. There are some specific drug interactions to watch for and other idiosyncrasies that warrant monitoring.

BONE LOSS

Menopause combined with treatment with aromatase inhibitors can cause calcium loss from bones. The management of osteoporosis in women with breast cancer does not differ from that of women without breast cancer. Adequate dietary intake of calcium (1200 mg/day) and vitamin D (400–800 IU), regular exercise, and avoidance of smoking are recommended. Monitoring with a bone density scan and treatment with bisphosphonates should be instituted as necessary. Drugs used to slow bone loss include bisphosphonates (such as alendronate [Fosamax]), raloxifene, and calcitonin. Monitoring of bone density before starting an AI and during treatment is important. Cholesterol-lowering drugs (statins) have been proven to help reduce the risk of heart disease and are being explored to prevent osteoporosis.

MENOPAUSAL SYMPTOMS

Antidepressant agents are sometimes used to treat menopause-related symptoms of depression or mood changes, and they have been shown to reduce hot flashes in some studies. Some antidepressants may interact in a negative way with hormonal therapy, however, reducing its potency and effectiveness. One antidepressant that is widely recommended for menopausal patients is venlafaxine (Effexor), which appears to have the least adverse effect on how hormonal therapy functions. Another antidepressant that has shown some benefit in this patient group is gabapentin (Neurontin). (See Chapter 5 for more information about various agents for control of hot flashes.) Avoiding spicy foods and hot beverages also helps reduce hot flashes. Wearing cotton clothing that is breathable and wearing layers so that the top layer can be shed if a woman is feeling too hot have been reported to help as well. In addition, vitamin E and clonidine, which are typically used for high blood pressure, can help to reduce hot flashes for some women.

Although it will rarely come up in your practice, 1% of individuals diagnosed with breast cancer are men. These patients commonly have hormone receptor-positive tumors and may, therefore, take hormonal therapy as well. They, too, may experience the same types of side effects as female patients, especially hot flashes and night sweats.

Some physicians opt to monitor the endometrial lining of the uterus (for women taking tamoxifen) by performing an annual transvaginal ultrasound. This is usually initiated when a patient presents with new vaginal bleeding or spotting. If the lining is noted to be thicker than normal, an endometrial biopsy may be obtained on an outpatient basis.

Thyroid function sometimes changes at menopause and causes depression. This problem may be relieved by appropriate thyroid hormone replacement therapy. Vaginal dryness and lack of libido are common complaints of patients who are taking hormonal therapy. Recommending vaginal lubricants (and offering samples in your office if you have any available) and discussing with the patient and her partner alternative ways to visually and physically stimulate her sexual urges are encouraged. Vaginal estradiol appears to be contraindicated in postmenopausal women who are taking adjuvant AIs[28] (see additional information in Chapter 5). As previously, patients are advised to not take any form of HRT once they have been diagnosed with breast cancer. Women who were previously taking HRT at the time of their diagnosis may experience the most discomfort in adjusting to hormonal therapy, as the latter treatment takes them 180 degrees from where their hormone levels were prior to diagnosis. If traditional vaginal lubricants do not provide the relief the patient needs, prescribing a vaginal hormonal cream may be considered; this course of action should be discussed with the patient's oncologist first, however.

Some patients may develop urogenital atrophy as a menopausal symptom. Treatment of this problem may require a referral to a gynecologist who specializes in treating genitourinary conditions. Encouraging patients to perform Kegel exercises has been shown to mitigate this problem for some women. Emptying the bladder frequently is also helpful.

Hair loss is an issue for some patients with breast cancer. As yet, no studies are available that have definitively proved whether taking any medications (such as Rogaine) can counteract this hair loss. Women who have not yet grown back their hair following chemotherapy may battle with this problem the most, because hormonal therapy appears to keep the hair from regenerating to the degree anticipated after chemotherapy.

Frequently Asked Questions

1. ***Can I take my hormonal therapy every other day to help reduce the side effects?***

   There are no studies to support taking hormonal therapy in this manner. How effective the drug is taking it every other day rather than daily has not been studied. It is better to discuss the side effects with your healthcare provider and request assistance with solutions to minimize these symptoms.

2. ***Will I ever be able to feel like myself again and not be dealing with these residual problems from my treatment?***

   For most breast cancer survivors, the answer is yes. Side effects can linger for various periods of time, but the majority of long-term side effects from chemotherapy, hormonal therapy, and surgery in particular do usually resolve themselves.

3. ***If I want to consider getting delayed reconstruction, can I do this or was I only a candidate at the time of original breast cancer surgery?***

   The majority of patients are candidates for reconstruction, including long after mastectomy surgery was performed. Those who have had inflammatory breast cancer are usually advised to wait several years after completion of treatment, however, due to risk of local recurrence. If a patient has a family history that is significant for cardiac disease or has a personal history that warrants discussion about possible risks of developing cardiac disease, the plastic surgeon who will be performing the reconstruction should be made aware of this. It may affect the selection of the vessels being used if free flap reconstruction is the type of surgery to be performed.

REFERENCES

1. Mock V. Exercise manages fatigue during breast cancer treatment: a randomized controlled trial. *Psycho-Oncology.* 2005;14:464–477.

2. Stricker CT, Drake D, Hoyer KA, Mock V. Evidence-based practice for fatigue management in adults with cancer: exercise as an intervention. *Oncol Nurs Forum.* 2004;31(5):963–976.
3. Rossouw JE, Anderson GL, Prentice RL, et al. Risks and benefits of estrogen plus progestin in healthy postmenopausal women: principal results from the Women's Health Initiative randomized controlled trial. *JAMA.* 2002;288(3):321–333.
4. Pandya KJ, Thummala AR, Griggs JJ, et al. Pilot study using gabapentin for tamoxifen-induced hot flashes in women with breast cancer. *Breast Cancer Res Treat.* 2004;83(1):87–89.
5. Van Patten CL, Olivotto IO, Chambers GK, et al. Effect of soy phytoestrogens on hot flashes in postmenopausal women with breast cancer: a randomized controlled trial. *J Clin Oncol.* 2002;20(6):1449–1455.
6. Altundag M, Altundag K, Cengiz M, et al. The field of radiation therapy may affect health-related quality of life in patients with operable breast cancer. *J Clin Oncol.* 2004;22(9):1765; author reply, 1765–1766.
7. Højris I, Andersen J, Overgaard M, Overgaard J. Late treatment-related morbidity in breast cancer patients randomized to postmastectomy radiotherapy and systemic treatment versus systemic treatment alone. *Acta Oncol.* 2000;39(3):355–372.
8. McQuestion M. Evidence-based skin care management in radiation therapy. *Semin Oncol Nurs.* 2006;22(3): 163–173.
9. Pommier P, Gomez F, Sunyach MP, D'Hombres A, Carrie C, Montbarbon X. Phase III randomized trial of *Calendula officinalis* compared with trolamine

for the prevention of acute dermatitis during irradiation for breast cancer. *J Clin Oncol.* 2004; 22(8): 1447–1453.
10. Højris I, Overgaard M, Christensen JJ, Overgaard J. Morbidity and mortality of ischaemic heart disease in high-risk breast-cancer patients after adjuvant postmastectomy systemic treatment with or without radiotherapy: analysis of DBCG 82b and 82c randomized trials. Radiotherapy Committee of the Danish Breast Cancer Cooperative Group. *Lancet.* 1999;354(9188): 1425–1430.
11. Allen AM, Prosnitz RG, Ten Haken RK, et al. Body mass index predicts the incidence of radiation pneumonitis in breast cancer patients. *Cancer J.* 2005;11(5): 390–398.
12. Meric F, Buchholz TA, Mirza NQ, et al. Long-term complications associated with breast-conservation surgery and radiotherapy. *Ann Surg Oncol.* 2002;9(6): 543–549.
13. Lind PA, Wennberg B, Gagliardi G, et al. ROC curves and evaluation of radiation-induced pulmonary toxicity in breast cancer. *Int J Radiat Oncol Biol Phys.* 2006; 64(3):765–770.
14. Lind PA, Marks LB, Hardenbergh PH, et al. Technical factors associated with radiation pneumonitis after local +/– regional radiation therapy for breast cancer. *Int J Radiat Oncol Biol Phys.* 2002;52(1):137–143.
15. Minor GI, Yashar CM, Spanos WJ Jr, et al. The relationship of radiation pneumonitis to treated lung volume in breast conservation therapy. *Breast J.* 2006; 12(1):48–52.
16. Cuzick J, Stewart H, Rutqvist L, et al. Cause-specific mortality in long-term survivors of breast cancer who

participated in trials of radiotherapy. *J Clin Oncol.* 1994;12(3):447–453.

17. Ragaz J, Olivotto IA, Spinelli JJ, et al. Locoregional radiation therapy in patients with high-risk breast cancer receiving adjuvant chemotherapy: 20-year results of the British Columbia randomized trial. *J Natl Cancer Inst.* 2005;97(2):116–126.
18. Coen JJ, Taghian AG, Kachnic LA, et al. Risk of lymphedema after regional nodal irradiation with breast conservation therapy. *Int J Radiat Oncol Biol Phys.* 2003;55(5):1209–1215.
19. Golshan M, Martin WJ, Dowlatshahi K. Sentinel lymph node biopsy lowers the rate of lymphedema when compared with standard axillary lymph node dissection. *Am Surg.* 2003;69(3):209–211; discussion 212.
20. Golshan M, Smith B. Prevention and management of arm lymphedema in the patient with breast cancer. *J Support Oncol.* 2006;4(8):381–386.
21. Hinrichs CS, Watroba NL, Rezaishiraz H, et al. Lymphedema secondary to postmastectomy radiation: incidence and risk factors. *Ann Surg Oncol.* 2004;11(6): 573–580.
22. Silberman AW, McVay C, Cohen JS, et al. Comparative morbidity of axillary lymph node dissection and the sentinel lymph node technique: implications for patients with breast cancer. *Ann Surg.* 2004;240(1):1–6.
23. Kocak Z, Overgaard J. Risk factors of arm lymphedema in breast cancer patients. *Acta Oncol.* 2000;39(3): 389–392.
24. Kligman L, Wong RK, Johnston M, et al. The treatment of lymphedema related to breast cancer: a systematic

review and evidence summary. *Support Care Cancer.* 2004;12(6):421–431.

25. Obedian E, Fischer DB, Haffty BG. Second malignancies after treatment of early-stage breast cancer: lumpectomy and radiation therapy versus mastectomy. *J Clin Oncol.* 2000;18(12):2406–2412.
26. Woodward WA, Strom EA, McNeese MD, et al. Cardiovascular death and second non-breast cancer malignancy after postmastectomy radiation and doxorubicin-based chemotherapy. *Int J Radiat Oncol Biol Phys.* 2003;57(2):327–335.
27. Galper S, Gelman R, Recht A, et al. Second nonbreast malignancies after conservative surgery and radiation therapy for early-stage breast cancer. *Int J Radiat Oncol Biol Phys.* 2002;52(2):406–414.
28. Kendall A, Dowestt M, Folkerd E, Smith I. Caution: vaginal estradiol appears to be contraindicated in postmenopausal women on adjuvant aromatase inhibitors. *Ann Oncol.* 2006;17(4):584–587.

CHAPTER 4

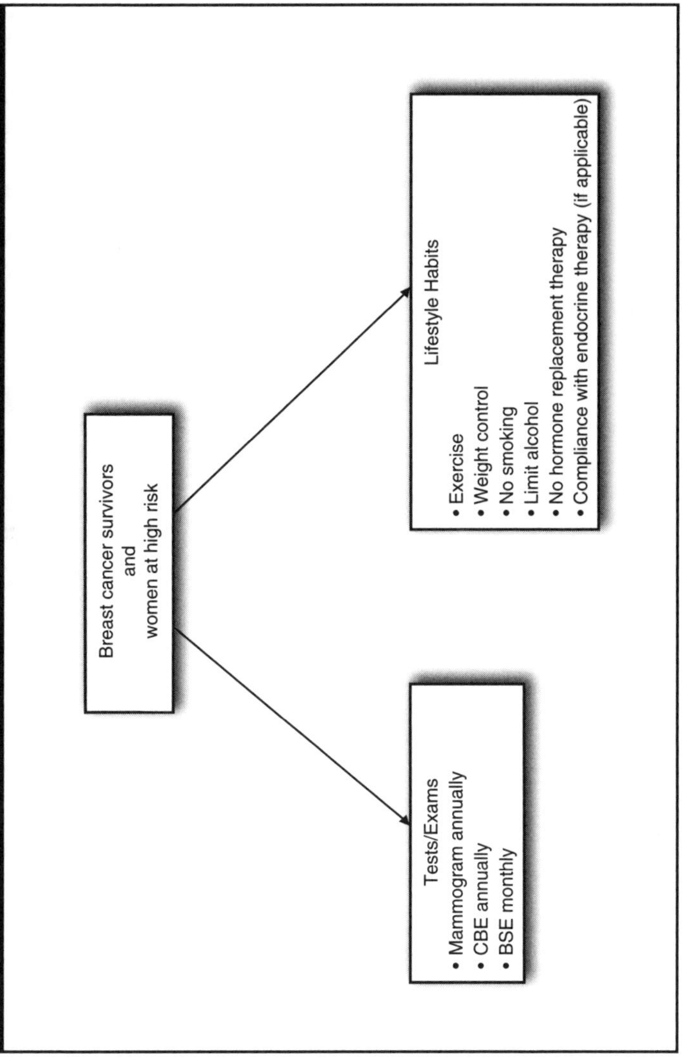

Algorithm for Promoting Compliance with Breast Health Care

CHAPTER 4

Promoting Compliance with Breast Health Care

Lillie D. Shockney, RN, BS, MAS

What you need to know:

Even women who have had breast cancer or who are at high risk for getting breast cancer may demonstrate nonadherence to health maintenance recommendations.

Women should be encouraged and routinely reminded of the importance of consistent breast health screening, including mammography, clinical breast examination (CBE), and breast self-examination (BSE).

Selecting a breast-imaging facility that provides results rapidly and offers easy access to appointments is important and helps promote compliance.

Each time you see your patient, check her chart to see when her next mammogram is due. Make sure she is comfortable performing a BSE. If she is not, arrange for someone to train her in the correct technique.

Promote healthy lifestyle habits to reduce risk. These include weight control, no smoking, and limited alcohol intake. If appropriate, refer your patient to a smoking-cessation program. Many excellent exercise programs for women are available that require a small time commitment on their part and that promote weight control and fitness. Contact the programs in your area and obtain a supply of their brochures for your office.

Hormonal therapy compliance remains an issue, despite well-documented studies demonstrating its effectiveness in the prevention of recurrence of disease in women who are breast cancer survivors as well as in the prevention of breast cancer in high-risk women. Ask your patient routinely if she is "taking her medications as prescribed" and inquire about any side effects she is experiencing that may deter her from taking the medication on a consistent basis. Talk with her oncologist, when appropriate, about whether additional measures can be taken to reduce side effects or about switching the patient to another form of hormonal therapy if necessary.

What your patient needs to know:

Annual mammography is important for early detection of breast cancer in at-risk women. Mammography, combined with annual clinical breast examinations (and in some cases semiannual examinations for women at risk) and monthly breast self-examinations, is the key to early detection and higher survival rates for women diagnosed with breast cancer and women at high risk of developing this disease.

If the patient is not confident about how to perform a breast self-examination, arrange for a nurse practitioner to teach her the correct technique. Most breast centers offer this service, so a referral should be easy to make.

This is a partnership you have with your patient when it comes to monitoring her breast health.

Lifestyle habits are tied to breast health. Specifically, obesity, smoking, and alcohol intake may increase the risk of getting breast cancer. Your patient needs to assume responsibility for watching her weight, avoiding smoking, and limiting alcohol consumption. If she needs help with any of these issues, she should make you aware so you can assist her. This may mean, for example, giving the patient a prescription for a smoking-cessation patch or advising her about what type of diet to follow or which exercise programs you believe are effective.

Hormonal therapy for breast cancer prevention or reduction of risk of recurrence is to be taken daily and at the prescribed dose. If the patient has side effects that prevent her from taking her medication as prescribed, she needs to bring this matter to your attention.

INTRODUCTION

There are two groups of patients—those who have had breast cancer or who have significant risk factors for getting this disease and those who do not. The ability to instill compliance in either group at times can be more challenging than anticipated. Although it might seem logical that someone who has had breast cancer would be fearful of recurrence and want to do everything in her power to prevent such a situation, as time goes on, the foxhole religion can seemingly wear off. As a result, these survivors may join the group of women who believe they are immune to breast cancer. No matter which group your patient falls into, promoting health is something we all try to encourage.

MAMMOGRAPHY

Excuses given by patients for not wanting to get a mammogram include pain from the procedure, fear of hearing bad results, lack of health insurance coverage, lack of time, belief that mammograms cause breast cancer, lack of faith that mammograms can detect cancer early, and the anxiety of waiting to get results if an abnormality is found on the screening mammogram. In reality, studies confirm that mammography saves lives (and saves breasts). As physicians, it is part of our responsibility to spread the facts and dispel the myths about mammography, because fear of the unknown is the worst fear of all.

Following are some ways to promote compliance with screening mammography:

- Refer patients to a breast imaging facility that provides results while the patient is there.
- Ensure easy access to appointments so patients can avoid time lost from work or other commitments.
- Emphasize the competence of the radiologist who is reading the images and the doctor who specializes in breast-imaging modalities.
- Identify efficiently run facilities so that patients' time spent there is as brief as possible.

- Educate patients about what the findings mean.
- Offer support services to help patients cope with a diagnosis of breast cancer.
- Provide timely feedback about the imaging results, and explain the next steps, if any are needed.
- Make appointments available immediately for women who do have a breast abnormality or abnormal screening mammogram and need diagnostic evaluation.

Ensuring that you are in the loop for getting the results promptly is also important, because your patients will rely on you for advice regarding the reported results.

Women whose health insurance does not cover screening mammograms may qualify for their state's breast and cervical screening program. These programs, which are available in every state and for which eligibility is based on specific financial criteria, can offer free screening. In addition, some institutions have obtained special grants that enable them to provide free transportation and even babysitting services, with the goal of encouraging even more women to come in for annual mammography. Your local health department and the American Cancer Society can provide you with information about these services. Studies have confirmed that providing a means of getting a free mammogram increases compliance.[1]

Although women continue to seek an "easier method" of breast imaging, mammography remains the gold standard for breast cancer detection today. Patients may hear stories about women whose cancer "was missed" on mammography, but it is important to reiterate to your patients at least once a year that most cancers are found at an early stage during annual mammograms.

Seek out a breast imaging facility for her that makes reminder phone calls a day in advance to tell patients that they are expected the next day for their mammogram. Reminding them of the location of the breast-imaging center and the time of their appointment helps to promote compliance and reduce no-show rates.

In addition, some healthcare providers reward their patients for compliance with health maintenance. Something as simple as a thank-you letter acknowledging that the patient did the right thing can be enough to promote future compliance.

CLINICAL BREAST EXAMINATION

There may be several opportunities to perform the annual clinical breast examination (CBE)—for example, at the time of the patient's annual gynecology appointment as well as when she sees her family doctor. Of course, having this opportunity requires the patient to adhere to the schedule of having an annual pelvic examination and physical examination. Take any opportunity that presents itself to perform the CBE, whether the patient is visiting her gynecologist for vaginitis or her primary care physician (PCP) for the flu. If her medical record shows that it has been 9 months or more since her last CBE, consider including it in the evaluation at that time. Contact her PCP and gynecologist and request that their offices send you copies of her clinic visits with them. This way you can see how often her breast health is being assessed by other providers.

BREAST SELF-EXAMINATION

When asked about breast self-examination (BSE), women often comment that they "don't know what they are supposed to be feeling for." Offering an instructional video, providing educational literature to take home including a shower card, and doing the examination with your patient will help her to understand the correct technique to use in performing this monthly exam. Although a patient may have many lumps and bumps, the goal is for her to learn what her "normal" is and to explore the breast tissue to see if there is something "new" since the last exam. Learning the geography of her breasts so she is comfortable with doing BSE is key. She should know to perform the exam a few days after her menstrual period ends or, if no longer menstruating, to select a day of the month that she will be consistently doing BSE. This will help BSE to become a habit as well as ensure that the breast tissue is at the same point in her menstrual cycle each time she does the evaluation.

It is important to reiterate that if the patient finds something during her BSE, it does not automatically mean that she has cancer. Most findings are benign. However, knowing when to call and who to call if she does find something can help ensure compliance.

Teaching young women how to do BSE beginning at age 21 can help the practice to become a health habit. It is a good idea to combine this education providing the facts about breast cancer and dispelling any myths that she may have heard that might instill more fear about the disease.

LIFESTYLE HABITS

There are several ways that a woman may be able to reduce her risk of getting breast cancer.

PHYSICAL ACTIVITY

Moderate activity for 30 minutes or more, 5 or more days per week, has been proven to help prevent breast cancer; exercising 3 to 5 hours per week demonstrated the greatest benefit in this regard. For prevention of breast cancer recurrence, it is recommended that patients engage in moderate activity for 30 minutes or more, 5 or more days per week; again, 3 to 5 hours of exercise per week is associated with the greatest benefit.[1]

WEIGHT CONTROL

Patients should consume a low-fat diet and watch their weight. Maintaining a body mass index (BMI) in the normal range for one's age group while increasing lean body mass has been found to be important in several respects:[2]

> Studies have shown that the risk of developing breast cancer is increased by 30% in postmenopausal women with BMIs exceeding 28 kg/m^2 compared to their counterparts with lower BMIs.[3] Premenopausal women with higher BMIs had a slightly lower risk.

> This difference in risk may reflect a decrease in circulating estrogens owing to the increased number of anovulatory cycles.
>
> In a prospective mortality study, the risk of recurrence of breast cancer increased with increasing BMI. There was a twofold increase in the risk of death for women with the highest BMIs (more than 40 kg/m^2) compared to those with the lowest BMIs (24.9 kg/m^2).[4]

SMOKING

All patients should avoid cigarette smoke—including secondary smoke. Smoking can be one of the hardest habits to break, because it will have become a nicotine addiction for some patients. It may be helpful to discuss steps to take to achieve smoking cessation with your patients and to describe what you can offer to help wean them off cigarettes (e.g., nicotine patches). This is an opportune time to discuss how smoking affects other health issues, such as cardiac disease, hypertension, and diabetes. Clearly, avoiding smoking has many benefits.[5]

ALCOHOL CONSUMPTION

Most women should limit their alcohol intake to one drink per day. An estimated 2% of breast cancers in the United States are attributed to alcohol intake; the mechanism underlying this etiology has been hypothesized to be direct DNA damage, alcohol's effects on hormone levels, or alcohol's effects on vitamin levels.[6] An adequate intake of folic acid (at least 400 mg/day) is needed to help offset the effect of moderate drinking (defined as one alcoholic beverage per day).

PROMOTING COMPLIANCE WITH HORMONAL THERAPY

For patients who are on long-term hormonal therapy for breast cancer prevention or to reduce their risk of breast cancer recurrence, the side effects of hormonal therapy can deter them from taking these medications as prescribed. Chapter 5 provides more information about this issue and suggestions on how you can increase your patients' compliance with their medication regimens.

ONGOING EDUCATION ABOUT BREAST CANCER

Patients may want to stay up to date on information published in credible medical journals related to discoveries associated with breast cancer risk reduction and prevention. This may be an area with which you can specifically help your patients. Consider providing consumer medical updates in your waiting room, sending periodic mailings to patients' homes, and alerting your patients to relevant educational programs offered in the community. As a way to promote breast health habits, some breast centers are partnering with local colleges to hold on-campus "Breastival" events, which are designed to educate college students about breast cancer and the active role they can play in reducing their risk. Some breast centers have partnered with local churches in an effort to reach underserved populations with their breast health message; this has also proven to be an effective way to promote compliance.

In addition, the American Cancer Society offers a free course through which laypersons can become breast health educators. This 3-hour course provides people with the tools needed to conduct a 30- or 60-minute program in their local community (for example, in parent–teacher associations and women's clubs) in which to promote screening mammography, CBE, and BSE. These programs can also provide facts and dispel myths about breast cancer and its treatment.

Frequently Asked Questions

1. ***What are the important components of breast health assessment?***

   The most important elements are the annual clinical breast examination, annual mammogram (for women beginning at age 40), and monthly breast self-examination.

2. ***Which lifestyle habits should be assessed that influence a woman's risk of getting breast cancer?***

   Risk factors for breast cancer include weight gain, smoking, excess alcohol intake, use of hormone replacement therapy (HRT), and sedentary lifestyle. Take the time to ask your patients about their exercise routine, evaluate their BMI, counsel them about not smoking (which affects the development of many other types of cancer as well as heart disease), and encourage them to limit their alcohol intake. Before prescribing HRT for any patient, you should weigh her risk of getting breast cancer against her desire to take HRT for control of menopausal symptoms.

3. ***What should I tell a patient who says that she does not know what she should look for when doing a breast self-examination?***

   Put your patient in touch with a trained nurse practitioner who routinely performs clinical breast examinations for instruction in the correct technique for doing a BSE. Encourage your patient to learn the geography of her breasts, and emphasize that lumps and bumps are not unusual. The important thing is to be able to identify a change in her breast geography from month to month. Encourage your patient to perform a BSE consistently at the same time each month.

REFERENCES

1. Phillips KA, Kerlikowske K, Baker LC, et al. Factors associated with women's adherence to mammography screening guidelines. *Health Serv Res.* 1998;33(1):29–53.
2. Irwin ML, McTiernan A, Bernstein L, et al. Relationship of obesity and physical activity with C-peptide, leptin, and insulin-like growth factors in breast cancer survivors. *Cancer Epidemiol Biomarkers Prev.* 2005;14(12):2881–2888.
3. Van den Brandt PA, Spiegelman D, Yaun SS, et al. Pooled analysis of prospective cohort studies on height, weight and breast cancer risk. *Am J Epidemiol.* 2000;152(6):514–527.

4. Calle EE, Rodriguez C, Walker-Thurmond K, Thun MJ. Overweight, obesity, and mortality from cancer in prospective studied cohort of US adults. *N Engl J Med.* 2003; 348(17):1625–1638.
5. Fentiman IS, Allen DS, Hamed H. Smoking and prognosis in women with breast cancer. *Int J Clin Pract.* 2005;59(9):1051–1054.
6. Smoth-Warner SA, Spiegelman D, Yaun SS, et al. Alcohol and breast cancer in women: a pooled analysis of cohort studies. *JAMA.* 1998;279(7):535–540.

CHAPTER 5

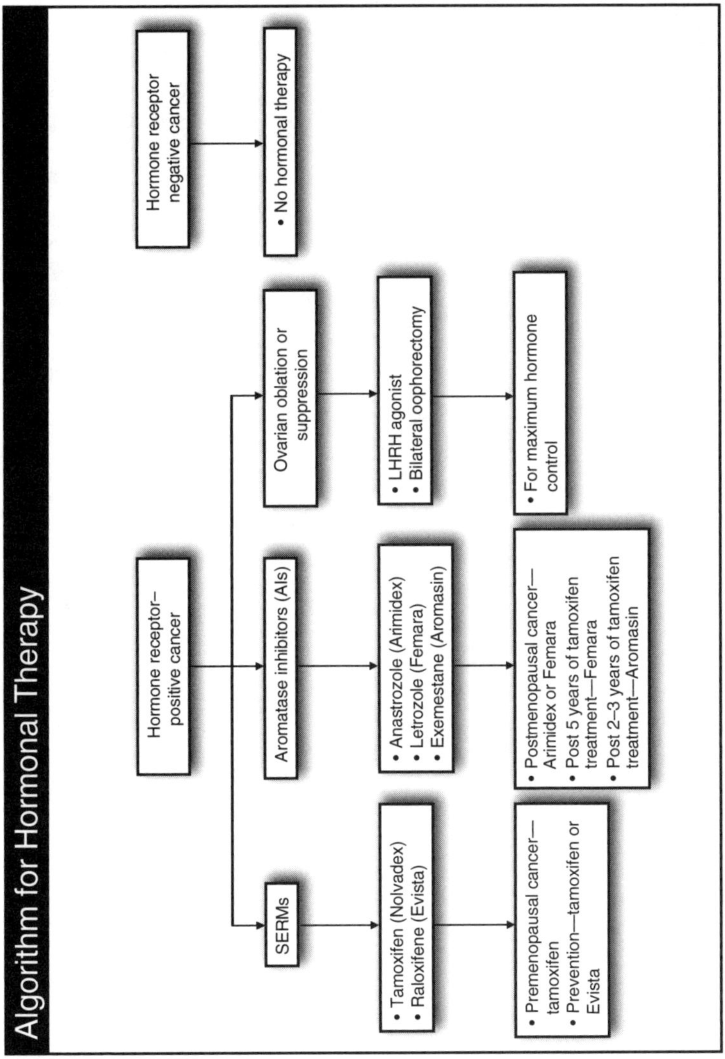
Algorithm for Hormonal Therapy
Hormone receptor–positive cancer
SERMs
Aromatase inhibitors (AIs)
Ovarian oblation or suppression
• Tamoxifen (Nolvadex)
• Raloxifene (Evista)
• Anastrozole (Arimidex)
• Letrozole (Femara)
• Exemestane (Aromasin)
• LHRH agonist
• Bilateral oophorectomy
• Premenopausal cancer—tamoxifen
• Prevention—tamoxifen or Evista
• Postmenopausal cancer—Arimidex or Femara
• Post 5 years of tamoxifen treatment—Femara
• Post 2–3 years of tamoxifen treatment—Aromasin
• For maximum hormone control
Hormone receptor negative cancer
• No hormonal therapy

CHAPTER 5

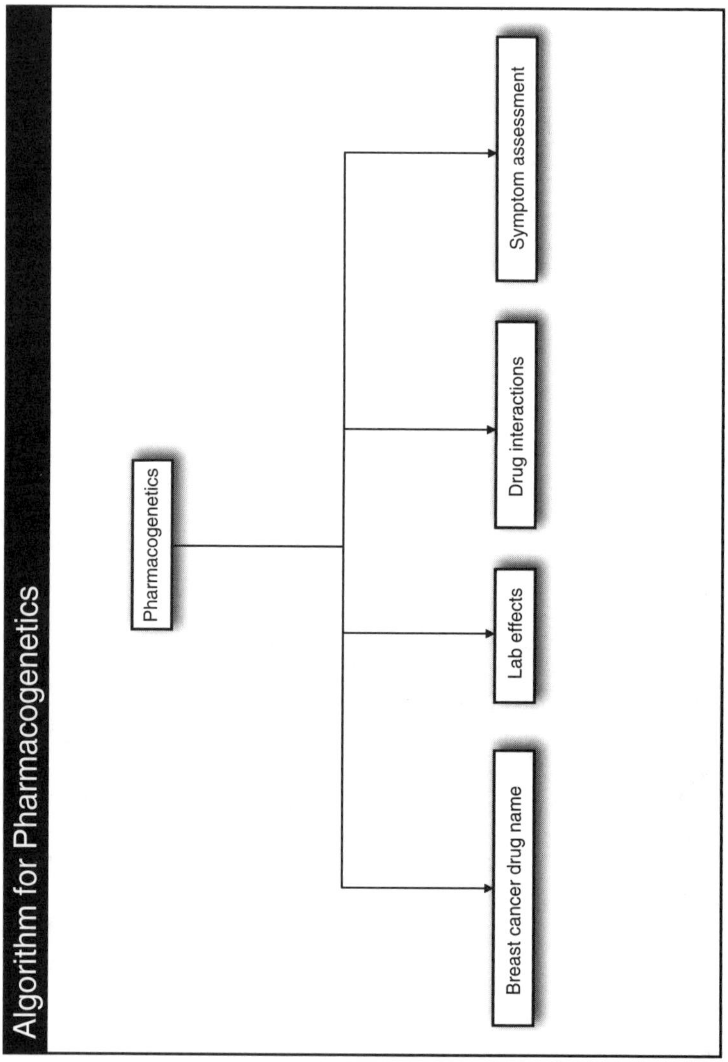
Algorithm for Pharmacogenetics
Pharmacogenetics
Breast cancer drug name
Lab effects
Drug interactions
Symptom assessment

CHAPTER 5

Hormonal Therapy and Pharmacogenetics

Lillie D. Shockney, RN, BS, MAS

HORMONAL THERAPY

What you need to know:

Approximately 50% of women are candidates for hormonal therapy and are advised to take it to prevent breast cancer recurrence. These women have tumors that are sensitive to estrogen (estrogen-receptor positive [ER1]) or progesterone (progesterone-receptor positive [PR1]) as determined by histopathologic evaluation.

Patient education is paramount for ensuring compliance with hormonal therapy. This is due in part to the need to take the drug for several years, combined with its many possible side effects, which may lead to frustration in some patients.

Each time you see your patient, you should ask her how she is doing on her hormonal therapy and reiterate this treatment's role in breast cancer prevention.

Premenopausal women are prescribed selective estrogen-receptor modulators (SERMs) and postmenopausal women are prescribed aromatase inhibitors (AIs). The only exception to this practice occurs with women who are diagnosed with ductal carcinoma in situ (DCIS). Women with DCIS, no matter what their menopausal status, are usually prescribed tamoxifen, a SERM.

The risk of uterine cancer and deep vein thrombosis (DVT), or both, from taking tamoxifen is extremely low. Nevertheless, many patients assume that their risk for these conditions is high. They need reassurance that this is not the case. Women who are usually advised not to take this drug are smokers and those with a previous history of DVT, transient ischemic attack, or stroke.

AIs can result in bone loss, so bone density tests are important for monitoring the bone health of patients who take these agents. You may prescribe bisphosphonates in such cases.

Because of estrogen depletion, cholesterol levels should also be monitored on a routine basis.

Patients should not take any form of hormone replacement therapy (HRT) if they are diagnosed with breast cancer. If a patient is taking HRT and receives this diagnosis, she needs to be weaned off the HRT soon after her diagnosis and must remain off of this medication, even if her tumor was hormone-receptor negative.

Educate your premenopausal patient about the importance of continuing some effective means of birth control even if she is not menstruating during hormonal therapy.

If your patient has limited finances, most drug companies provide a discounted program for obtaining the hormonal therapy agents they manufacture.

Ovarian ablation or suppression is used for BRCA1- or BRCA2-positive patients to prevent breast cancer as well as ovarian cancer. It is also used as a means of providing maximum hormonal control.

Hormonal therapy (SERMs) may also be prescribed for women who are at a high risk of developing breast cancer—those with a significant family history or who are positive for the BRCA1 or BRCA2 gene—and have elected to not have preventive mastectomy surgery.

What your patient needs to know:

Women who have tumors that are hormone-receptor positive are commonly advised to take hormonal therapy. Hormonal therapy is not to be confused with HRT. In fact, the patient should actually think of the two as being polar opposites.

Approximately 50% of women who are diagnosed with breast cancer will be advised to take hormonal therapy. Hormonal therapy is also prescribed to high-risk women as a means of preventing breast cancer.

It is extremely important to take the medication as prescribed. If the patient is experiencing side effects that are affecting her quality of life, she needs to notify her oncologist and discuss methods to reduce these side effects with the goal of maintaining her on hormonal therapy.

Even if a woman no longer has her ovaries, her body can still manufacture estrogen through her adrenal glands. She also stores estrogen in her body fat.

Women who have been diagnosed with breast cancer should not take any form of HRT. This group includes women whose breast cancer was hormone-receptor negative.

Menopausal symptoms are the most common symptoms reported with HRT. If these symptoms are severe, doctors can recommend drugs and methods to reduce these side effects.

Patients have a tendency to want to jump from one form of hormonal therapy to another in hopes of experiencing fewer and less severe side effects. No data have been collected on the effect of switching therapies in this way from the perspective of risk reduction. Women commonly ask for the hormonal therapy with the least side effects rather than asking which hormonal therapy is the most effective for the particular clinical situation.

Women may experience other medical problems as a result of taking hormonal therapy, including bone loss when taking an AI. Regular exercise and calcium intake are recommended for patients who take AIs. In some cases, patients may be advised to take a prescription bone-building agent. Cholesterol elevation may also be an issue when taking AIs, so it important for the patient to watch her fat intake and for her doctor to monitor her blood levels on a routine basis.

Most women assume that tamoxifen will cause uterine cancer and/or stroke. The incidence of these serious complications is actually very low. Women taking this drug should not smoke, however.

Hormonal therapy is taken for several years. Thus the patient needs to make a commitment to herself and to her doctors that she will be compliant in taking the medication daily and at the recommended dose.

INTRODUCTION

Nonadherence with prescribed medication is an age-old problem. Despite the ability of medicines to prevent, relieve, and even cure many types of illness, people often do not take them as prescribed.[1] The potential to improve health outcomes through better compliance with therapy represents an enormous opportunity in terms of both reducing patient burden and decreasing the cost of disease management.

Studies that have been conducted by various pharmaceutical companies based on interviews with oncologists have found that most doctors believe their patients are compliant in taking their medications as prescribed.[2] The data from the patients, however, tell a different story. Awareness of this problem may be the first critical step in improving adherence to maintain optimal health. Despite the fact that breast cancer is a serious disease, patients do not always take their medications as prescribed. As former Surgeon General C. Everett Koop stated, "Drugs don't work in patients who don't take them."[3]

A large percentage (50%) of breast cancer patients are advised to take hormonal therapy after completing their breast cancer treatment of surgery, chemotherapy, and/or radiation therapy. Today, hormonal therapy commonly is prescribed for many consecutive years—even as long as a decade. During this posttreatment phase, patients are seen less often by their oncology healthcare providers, but it is hoped they will periodically keep their primary care provider (PCP), gynecologist, and other healthcare practitioners involved in maintaining their general health and well-being. This makes your role as a healthcare provider for these patients increasingly important, as you will have the opportunity to promote compliance with hormonal therapy during these patient encounters. Levels of patient compliance with medications are not definitively known, even though compliance with hormonal therapy may influence its effectiveness as a means of breast cancer prevention.

The depth and content of patient education given to breast cancer survivors about the purpose of taking hormonal therapy, importance of compliance with the dose and frequency, and management of potential side effects vary among providers. Patients may not voluntarily tell their healthcare providers that they are not taking their medications as prescribed. This lack of compliance may be due to not understanding the importance of the drug regimen, unwillingness to cope with side effects that affect quality of life for a long period, or even embarrassment about reporting this information (e.g., sexual side effects, menopausal symptoms, lack of financial resources to purchase the medication). Clinical studies rely on, and to some degree assume, patient compliance when measuring efficacy of the drug therapy; however, compliance with self-administration of drugs is not one of the elements measured and assessed as part of most hormonal therapy outcomes studies.

This section begins with an overview of hormonal therapy and then discusses the potential side effects that can cause patients to not comply with the recommended medication regimen. The chapter also provides information about ways to reduce the side effects associated with hormonal therapy and suggests when to consider recommending that a patient contact her oncologist to discuss the hormonal therapy plan.

There is also information regarding drugs that may interfere with the metabolism and effectiveness of the hormonal therapy she is taking.

TYPES OF HORMONAL THERAPY

There are two categories of hormonal therapy: selective estrogen-receptor modulators (SERMs) and aromatase inhibitors (AIs). In recent years, results of studies have been published—with still more research currently under way—demonstrating the benefit of these medications in preventing recurrence of disease.

Selective Estrogen-Receptor Modulators

SERMs are prescribed to treat both premenopausal women and postmenopausal women who have noninvasive early or advanced disease (e.g., DCIS). These drugs are also approved for women who are considered to be at high risk for breast cancer even though they lack a personal history of the disease.

SERMs act on some parts of the body (such as bones) much like estrogen does and help prevent bone loss as a woman ages. They do not have estrogen-like effects on other parts of the body, however. This class of drugs works by binding (attaching) to estrogen receptors and selectively modulating the effects of estrogen in different body tissues. Because not all estrogen receptors are the same, these differences allow SERMs to have one effect in one kind of tissue and a different effect in another kind of tissue.

Tamoxifen (Nolvadex), a synthetic drug used in breast cancer prevention and treatment, was the first SERM developed and has the longest track record for use as hormonal therapy for breast cancer. It was considered the gold standard for breast cancer treatment for more than 20 years. This drug blocks the effects of estrogen on the breast and has been shown to reduce the risk of cancer recurrence as well as to prevent cancer from developing in the other (contralateral) breast. Side effects of tamoxifen include an increased risk of certain visual disturbances, fatal pulmonary embolism, and cancer of both the endometrium and the body of the uterus. The antiestrogenic effects of tamoxifen on breast cells appear to reverse after 5 years; the drug may then become cancer promoting, for reasons that are not clear. Tamoxifen has been proven to reduce the risk of breast cancer by 47%.[4]

Raloxifene (Evista) was the second synthetic SERM to reach the market, and it is similar in some ways to tamoxifen. It is currently prescribed to protect women against osteoporosis and heart disease without increasing their risk for breast cancer. However, it does not protect bones as well as estrogen does. The results of the Study of Tamoxifen and Raloxifene Trial (STAR) have confirmed that raloxifene is as effective as tamoxifen in breast cancer prevention and may be associated with slightly fewer side effects that are worrisome to some patients, potentially resulting in a higher level of compliance with the therapy.

Other SERMs are currently being developed. Ideally, a SERM would have all the benefits of estrogen but none of the risks. No SERM is as yet available in the United States that meets those criteria, but research is under way with that goal in mind.

Common side effects of tamoxifen include hot flashes, vaginal discharge or bleeding, and menstrual irregularities. Some women also experience hair loss or skin rashes when taking this drug.

Although the complication is uncommon (less than 1% incidence), women who take tamoxifen are at increased risk of developing blood clots in their lungs and legs. These women also have a small risk of developing two different types of uterine cancer. If a patient is taking tamoxifen and experiences any sudden chest pain, shortness of breath, coughing up blood, pain or swelling in her legs, or vaginal bleeding, she should seek medical help immediately. Women taking tamoxifen should not smoke, because this behavior increases their risk of DVT and/or stroke.

Aromatase Inhibitors

AIs reduce the levels of estrogen in the body. Anastrozole (Arimidex), letrozole (Femara), and exemestane (Aromasin) are three such synthetic hormones approved by the U.S. Food and Drug Administration (FDA) for treating advanced breast cancer. Both anastrozole and letrozole have also received FDA approval for use as adjuvant therapy in early-stage breast cancer. All three of these agents are very potent drugs and can produce a marked reduction in estrogen levels.

The main source of estrogen for premenopausal women is the ovaries. When women enter menopause, their ovaries stop producing estrogen, but estrogen levels do not drop off completely. Estrogen is still present from another process in the body—the conversion of a substance from women's adrenal glands into estrogen. Specifically, this substance, androstenedione, circulates through the body to tissues such as muscle, fat, and even breast cancers themselves, where it is converted to estrogen.

The conversion of androstenedione to estrogen is driven by an enzyme called aromatase; AIs stop this conversion process. These agents differ from tamoxifen in that they actually reduce the amount of estrogen in the body. Tamoxifen, by contrast, blocks the effects of estrogen in the body by competing with estrogen for the estrogen receptor—the receptor to which estrogen binds so as to exert its effect.

Side effects associated with AIs are generally mild. In recent clinical trials with these agents, women reported hot flashes, joint pain, and muscle aches as the most bothersome side effects.

However, a major concern with AIs is the fact that they lower the body's estrogen level, which may put the patient at a higher risk for osteoporosis. If your patient is taking an AI in the adjuvant (or any other) setting, be aware of the potential for osteoporosis and the need to monitor her bone mineral density.

Lower estrogen levels in the body also affect blood lipid levels. For this reason, some doctors are concerned that AIs might increase the risk of heart problems or cardiovascular disease.

Because there are more than 30 years of research and experience with tamoxifen but a relatively brief period of experience with AIs, other side effects associated with AIs might potentially be discovered that will warrant further investigation.

STUDY RESULTS

The Arimidex/tamoxifen, alone or in combination (ATAC) trial compared tamoxifen with anastrozole as the treatment given after the removal of breast cancer. This large clinical trial evaluated the use of anastrozole as adjuvant therapy for 5 years in postmenopausal women with localized hormone receptor-positive breast cancer. In this study, the investigators found that women who were taking anastrozole were less likely to experience a breast cancer recurrence than were the women taking tamoxifen.

This study raised an important point: the need to confirm that a woman is postmenopausal by performing blood tests rather than by relying solely on whether she has been menstruating, because chemotherapy often results in a discontinuation in menses during and sometimes for several months after treatment. The patient's hormone levels, however, may signal that she still is premenopausal or perimenopausal.

The FDA has approved the use of anastrozole as an adjuvant therapy option only for postmenopausal women. The results from the ATAC trial suggest that the best treatment option for postmenopausal women with hormone receptor-positive breast cancer is to bypass tamoxifen and start out immediately with 5 years of anastrozole as adjuvant therapy.

A second clinical trial looked into a possible next step after tamoxifen therapy. Researchers evaluated the use of letrozole (another AI) after 5 years of tamoxifen use in postmenopausal women who had been treated for breast cancer. Most experts believe that 5 years of tamoxifen treatment for early breast cancer is the optimal duration; tamoxifen therapy that lasts for more than 5 years does not improve outcomes and, in fact, may be harmful. Indeed, increased rates of the serious complications of uterine cancer and DVT have been reported with increased duration of tamoxifen therapy.[5]

Study results have shown that letrozole, when given after tamoxifen, reduces the risk of breast cancer recurrence by almost half. Thus letrozole provides a new extended adjuvant treatment option for women who have completed 5 years of tamoxifen therapy. The decision to use letrozole will be based on a number of factors, including an estimate of the patient's remaining risk of developing breast cancer.[6]

Results from a third clinical trial indicate that, rather than the patient taking tamoxifen for 5 years, it may be better to switch her to an AI after 2 to 3 years of tamoxifen therapy. This trial, which was called the Intergroup Exemestane Study, randomized women who had already taken tamoxifen for 2 to 3 years to one of two groups: (1) a group that completed the 5-year course of tamoxifen, or (2) a group that switched to exemestane (an AI) to complete a total of 5 years of hormonal treatment.

This study demonstrated that the women who switched to exemestane had almost a one-third reduction in risk of recurrence of breast cancer, compared with women who remained on tamoxifen. Cancers in the opposite (contralateral) breast were also reduced by more than half in the women who switched to exemestane. Researchers concluded that women who elect to start tamoxifen appear to benefit from switching to exemestane after 2 to 3 years, rather than waiting until they have completed the full 5-year course of tamoxifen therapy.[7]

The findings from all three of these studies apply only to women who are postmenopausal. No benefits from AIs have been shown in women who are still having menstrual periods.

A great deal of debate has focused on the role of AIs in early-stage breast cancer. In 2006, the American Society of Clinical Oncology (ASCO) convened an expert panel to examine all of the available data related to this issue. The ASCO panel recommended that optimal adjuvant hormonal therapy for postmenopausal women with receptor-positive breast cancer include an AI as initial therapy or after treatment with tamoxifen. The panel further recommended that each woman and her doctor weigh the risks and benefits of all potential therapies based on the patient's individual circumstances.

CONTROLLING SIDE EFFECTS

Antidepressant agents are sometimes used to treat menopause-related symptoms of depression or mood changes, and they have been shown to reduce hot flashes in some studies. Some antidepressants may interact in a negative way with hormonal therapy, however, reducing its potency and effectiveness. One antidepressant that is widely recommended for menopausal patients is venlafaxine (Effexor), which appears to have the least adverse effect on how hormonal therapy functions. Another antidepressant that has shown some benefit in this patient group is gabapentin (Neurontin). A study comparing various agents for control of hot flashes provided the information shown in Table 5-1 regarding centrally active hormonal hot flash therapies.[8]

Avoiding spicy foods and hot beverages also helps reduce hot flashes. Wearing cotton clothing that is breathable, and wearing layers so that the top layer can be shed if a woman is feeling too hot, have been reported to help as well. In addition, vitamin E and clonidine, which are typically used for high blood pressure, can help to reduce hot flashes for some women.

TABLE 5-1 Agents for Potential Control of Hot Flashes

Drug Name	Dosage	Observed Reduction	Side Effects
Bellergal	2 pills/day	Slight	Increased dry mouth, dizziness
Clonidine	0.1 mg/day (transdermal)	Significant	Increased dry mouth, difficulty sleeping, constipation, drowsiness
Methyldopa	250 mg/day	Significant	Increased fatigue, weakness, dizziness, nausea
Venlafaxine	75 mg/day	Significant	Increased dry mouth, sleeplessness, decreased appetite
Paroxetine	25 mg/day	Significant	None

Although it will rarely come up in your practice, 1% of individuals diagnosed with breast cancer are men. These patients commonly have hormone-receptor-positive tumors and may, therefore, take hormonal therapy as well. They, too, may experience the same types of side effects as female patients, especially hot flashes and night sweats.

Some physicians opt to monitor the endometrial lining of the uterus (for women taking tamoxifen) by performing an annual transvaginal ultrasound. This is usually initiated when a patient presents with new vaginal bleeding or spotting. If the lining is noted to be thicker than normal, an endometrial biopsy may be obtained on an outpatient basis.

Thyroid function sometimes changes at menopause and causes depression. This problem may be relieved by appropriate thyroid hormone replacement therapy.

Drugs used to slow bone loss include bisphosphonates (such as alendronate [Fosamax]), raloxifene, and calcitonin. Monitoring of bone density before starting an AI and during treatment is important. Cholesterol-lowering drugs called statins have been proven to help reduce the risk of heart disease and are being explored to prevent osteoporosis.

Vaginal dryness and lack of libido are common complaints of patients who are taking hormonal therapy. Recommending vaginal lubricants (and offering samples in your office if you have any available) and discussing with the patient and her partner alternative ways to visually and physically stimulate her sexual urges are encouraged. Vaginal estradiol appears to be contraindicated in postmenopausal women who are taking adjuvant AIs.[9]

As previously, patients are advised to not take any form of HRT once they have been diagnosed with breast cancer. Women who were previously taking HRT at the time of their diagnosis may experience the most discomfort in adjusting to hormonal therapy, as the latter treatment takes them 180 degrees from where their hormone levels were prior to diagnosis. If traditional vaginal lubricants do not provide the relief the patient needs, prescribing a vaginal hormonal cream may be considered; this course of action should be discussed with the patient's oncologist first, however.

Some patients may already be on an antidepressant for treatment of clinical depression. Others may be advised to take an antidepressant to help control their hot flashes and night sweats. Refer to the pharmacogenetics section for more details about drug interactions to be aware of. There are a number of antidepressants, and whether they are strong, moderate, or weak (or no effect) inhibitors of the enzyme CYP2D6 is a potential marker of whether they can effect the metabolism of tamoxifen. Antidepressants with the least impact with interfering with tamoxifen are Effexor and Lexapro.

Some patients may develop urogenital atrophy as a menopausal symptom. Treatment of this problem may require a referral to a gynecologist who specializes in treating genitourinary conditions. Encouraging patients to perform Kegel exercises has been shown to mitigate this problem for some women. Emptying the bladder frequently is also helpful.

Hair loss is an issue for some patients with breast cancer. As yet, no studies are available that have definitively proved whether taking any medications (such as Rogaine) can counteract this hair loss. Women who have not yet grown back their hair following chemotherapy may battle with this problem the most, because hormonal therapy appears to keep the hair from regenerating to the degree anticipated after chemotherapy.

BIRTH CONTROL

Some women assume that if they are not menstruating, they cannot conceive. It is important to reiterate to your patient that it remains critically important to practice birth control while taking SERMs because it has not been determined that she is truly postmenopausal. SERMs can produce serious congenital anomalies so they should not be used in fertile women.

PROMOTING COMPLIANCE WITH HORMONAL THERAPY

There is a lot of information on the Internet—some helpful and some not. It is common to find breast cancer patients who are actively seeking information through this easy-to-access resource and who may shy away from taking hormonal therapy owing to fears of the side effects described by other patients. Patients should be encouraged to rely on their healthcare team rather than an online chat room, where misinformation—rather than evidenced-based results—may be disseminated.

Factors that influence patients' compliance with therapy have been studied. These factors include prolonged administration of the medication, side effects, poor understanding of the need for the drug and its purpose, psychological issues, cost, and low motivation. A common finding has been that patients do not understand that their disease is serious enough to warrant this additional treatment.[10]

Because there is a high likelihood that patients will see you more often than they see their oncology doctors and nurses, oncologists rely on professionals like yourself to promote compliance with hormonal therapy. When you speak with your patients, consider discussing these issues using the following format:

> Your oncologist has prescribed hormonal therapy [drug name] for you as a way to help prevent recurrence of your breast cancer. This is a long-term therapy that you will take for several years. I want to help you if you are experiencing any issues related to taking this medication. So fill me in on how you are doing:
>
> 1. Are you taking your hormonal therapy as prescribed?
> 2. Are you experiencing any side effects that are affecting your quality of life?
> 3. Have you discussed these side effects with your prescribing oncologist and, if so, how long ago did this discussion take place?
> 4. Are you experiencing any sexual side effects that we can discuss today and find solutions for?

5. Do you have a prescription plan to cover the expenses of this medication?
6. I would like to talk with your medical oncologist about the side effects that you are having so that we might together decide on some remedies for you.

Because hormonal therapy requires a long-term commitment on the part of the patient, it falls into the same category as many other medications that are used to treat chronic illnesses. With all of these medications, problems with compliance may arise over time.

Here are some additional strategies to reinforce or improve adherence with hormonal therapy:

1. All healthcare providers involved with the patient's care should be made aware of the issues and importance of adherence to this medication regimen.
2. Monitor the patient's compliance with her medication during each office visit. If she misses an appointment, call and inquire about her compliance.
3. Identify patients who may be at higher risk for noncompliance, and provide additional monitoring steps to help ensure that they are taking their medications as prescribed.
4. Encourage the patient to report side effects and work with her to manage those side effects. This step may require a call to her oncologist to obtain more information about what is safe to prescribe in the patient's particular circumstances.

5. Keep the patient informed about research results associated with hormonal therapy so that she is an informed patient. This conversation may also serve as a catalyst for the patient to discuss any issues she has about continuing to take the medication as prescribed.

6. Assess the patient's financial situation to ensure that she can afford the medications. If cost is an issue, there are financial resources available through most of the pharmaceutical companies to offset the expense of the drug. (See the Resources of Benefit section at the end of this book for more information.)

OVARIAN ABLATION OR SUPPRESSION

In recent years, the role of ovarian ablation as a therapeutic modality in both the prevention and the treatment of breast cancer has resurfaced, long after its earliest use for this purpose nearly a century ago. Bilateral oophorectomy has proved effective in reducing the risk of developing breast cancer for women who are both BRCA1 and BRCA2 carriers. Tamoxifen reduces the risk of breast cancer for BRCA2 carriers but not for BRCA1 carriers.[11]

For premenopausal women with ER-positive tumors, a second option is endocrine therapy, which aims to suppress mitogenic estrogen signaling. Until recently, 5 years of tamoxifen therapy was regarded as the standard adjuvant endocrine therapy. Ovarian ablation is also effective in treating premenopausal women and can be achieved by surgery, radiation, or the use of a luteinizing hormone-releasing hormone (LHRH) analog such as goserelin. The tamoxifen/goserelin combination provides more effective estrogen blocking than use of either drug alone. However, given that the third generation of AIs has demonstrated improved efficacy over tamoxifen in postmenopausal women with early- or advanced-stage disease, combination treatment with goserelin plus an AI may also provide optimal blocking in premenopausal women.[12]

Although ovarian ablation is an effective adjuvant therapy for primary breast cancer, little is understood about its effect on quality of life compared with the more widely used adjuvant chemotherapy. For some women, preserving ovarian function is a priority for the future, particularly if they have not yet had a family. For premenopausal patients in whom estrogen synthesis occurs primarily in the ovaries, treatment options may include ovarian ablation or suppression along with hormonal therapy. Although some studies have demonstrated that ovarian ablation results in an outcome equivalent to that achieved with chemotherapy alone, studies examining the combination therapy have not demonstrated a clear benefit with the addition of ovarian suppression to standard chemotherapy.[13]

PHARMACOGENETICS

What you need to know:

Women do not always realize that other medications, herbs, and supplements they are taking may interfere with the drugs and therapies being given to them as part of their breast cancer treatment. Ask the patient about every drug, supplement, and vitamin she is taking; this is important baseline information to have for her medical record.

Patients will commonly ask their gynecologist, primary care provider (PCP), or you for "symptom relief" from drug side effects they are experiencing that are associated with hormonal therapy for breast cancer prevention or gastrointestinal side effects associated with chemotherapy or other drugs prescribed during their breast cancer treatment. Caution needs to be exercised before prescribing medications or even herbal options for these patients, as there may be contraindications to doing so.

What your patient needs to know:

Taking medications or herbal supplements without informing her healthcare providers is unwise for a breast cancer patient or survivor. Self-prescribing for symptom relief is also to be discouraged.

The patient should inform her doctor if she is having unpleasant side effects from a specific treatment so that he or she can appropriately prescribe something to help alleviate those side effects or direct the patient in another manner (such as exercising to counteract fatigue from radiation) to obtain symptom relief.

Some medications stay in the body for a long time. The patient needs to factor this in when considering adding other medications or supplements to her daily care program after she has completed a specific treatment regimen for her breast cancer.

OVERVIEW

The purpose of this section is to provide information related to breast cancer drugs that a patient is currently taking and that may result in side effects, complications, or reduction in effectiveness if given with other prescription medications or supplements. Before beginning, however, some background information on the science of pharmacogenetics is provided here.

Pharmacogenetics is the study of how the actions of and reactions to drugs vary with the patient's genes, and specifically how people respond to drug therapies. Although this science is still considered fairly new, there have already been many useful discoveries. It has long been known that genes influence the risk of developing certain diseases, and that genes determine traits such as hair and eye color. Genes can also alter the risk for developing different diseases. In more recent years, research has discovered that genes can determine other aspects of the individual, down to the level of the enzymes produced in the liver. Because these enzymes determine how quickly a drug is excreted from the body, they can make major differences in the way people respond to drugs. Some of the most basic work concerns the way race and gender influence drug reactions—and race and gender are genetically determined. More specific research has identified individual genes that may influence drug response and drug interactions. Specific genes have been identified that may determine how patients will respond to specific drugs.

CAUSES AND SYMPTOMS

Genes alter responses to drugs because genes influence many parts of the body itself. For example, in the case of gender-related responses to antidepressant agents, women tend to show greater responses to serotonin-specific antidepressants because women naturally have lower levels of serotonin than men do. This makes women more likely to develop a type of depression marked by low serotonin levels, but it also means that women will respond better to replacement of serotonin.

Another trait that is influenced by genes is the production of a liver enzyme, CYP2D6. This enzyme metabolizes some drugs by converting them to a form that can be removed from the body. Genes determine the level of this enzyme in the liver. People with low levels of CYP2D6 will metabolize drugs slowly. Slow metabolism means the drugs will act for a longer period of time. Slow metabolizers respond to smaller doses of medications that are eliminated by this enzyme, whereas fast metabolizers—that is, people who have a lot of the enzyme—will need larger drug doses to get the same effects. At the same time, low levels of CYP2D6 mean that people taking the drugs that are metabolized by this enzyme will have higher drug levels and are more likely to experience undesired side effects.

Yet another mechanism of drug activity is the presence or absence of specific drug receptor sites. Drugs act by binding to specific chemicals, called receptor sites, within body cells. Genes may help determine how many of these cells there are. Other genetic studies indicate that genes may affect how people respond to foods as well as to drugs. An Australian study of osteoporosis, for example, reported that separate genes may affect a person's response to vitamin D, calcium, and estrogens.

IMPLICATIONS

Although studies in the field of pharmacogenetics promise to provide great benefits in drug effectiveness and safety, at the present time most drug treatment involves trial and error. That is, the physician prescribes a medication, and the patient takes the drug in good faith assuming that it will help whatever problem the drug is designed to medically address. The drug may work, or it may not. It may cause adverse effects, or it may be safe. If the drug does not work, the dose is increased. If the drug causes harmful or undesired side effects, a new drug might be tried until, finally, the right drug is found. In some cases, this process may take weeks or even months. In the case of cancer therapies, there may not be another drug to which to switch the patient, thereby creating the challenge of how to manage the side effects so the patient can reap the benefits of cancer therapy.

Table 5-2 provides a list of the drug therapies most commonly given to breast cancer survivors and women at high risk for breast cancer. These drugs are in the classification of hormonal therapies. Drugs that the patient received during her chemotherapy treatment are not included as the effect of these medications should no longer be of active concern from a pharmacogenetics perspective. Table 5-2 lists the name of each drug, the class of the drug, the

TABLE 5-2 Hormonal Therapy Drugs and Their Interactions

Drug Name	Class	Lab Effects/ Interference	Drug Interactions
Exemestane (Aromasin)	Steroidal aromatase inhibitor	Lymphopenia (20% incidence) Elevated LFT (AST, ALT, alkaline phosphatase, GGT) rarely	CYP450 inducers: may increase drug clearance
Fulvestrant (Faslodex)	Estrogen-receptor downregulator	None	Currently unknown
Letrozole (Femara)	Nonsteroidal aromatase inhibitor	Liver transaminases may be transiently elevated	Currently unknown
Tamoxifen citrate (Nolvadex, Soltamox)	Antiestrogen	Decreased CBC Increased LFT and calcium levels Interference in lab tests as TFT and hyperlipidemia	Anticoagulants: increase PT; monitor PT closely and reduce anticoagulant dose CYP450 inhibitors and inducers: alter tamoxifen metabolism
Toremifene citrate (Fareston)	Synthetic tamoxifen analog	Decreased WBC and platelets	Testosterone and cyclosporine: may inhibit metabolism CYP450 inhibitors, and inducers alter tamoxifen metabolism

laboratory tests that are used to monitor the patient while taking that specific medication, and any medications, herbs, or supplements that are contraindicated while the patient is taking the therapy.

Frequently Asked Questions

1. ***If a patient is taking hormone replacement therapy and is newly diagnosed with breast cancer, what instructions should she be given about coming off this drug?***

   What usually works best is having the patient wean off the medication. The "cold turkey" approach can be emotionally distressing, especially when added to a new diagnosis of breast cancer. The patient needs to begin by taking the medication every other day, then every third day, then twice a week, and so on, until the drug is discontinued. Remember that her cancer did not form overnight, so the medication should be stopped gradually, too. It is necessary to stop hormone replacement therapy in case of breast cancer, but this weaning should be accomplished over a 2- to 3-week period.

2. ***Who is responsible for monitoring my patient's blood work while she is taking cancer medications that may affect her blood levels?***

   The doctor who prescribed the medications should be in charge of monitoring blood work the majority of the time; this provider is generally the patient's oncologist. However, if the patient is seeing you for a checkup or new onset of symptoms of some kind, it is appropriate to check her blood levels and contact her oncologist to make him or her aware of the results, whether they are abnormal or not.

3. ***If the chart provided says there are no known drug interactions, is it safe to assume that whatever I might prescribe for the patient will not negatively affect her treatment?***

   Although that would be the hope, research is ongoing in this area; therefore, it is prudent to stay abreast of updated reports that relate to the study of these drugs so that you will be aware of any new information that might affect your prescribing practices.

CHAPTER SUMMARY

Studies are under way at Johns Hopkins to better understand the barriers patients are experiencing that result in them choosing to not take their medication daily at the recommended dose. Some of these barriers include physical side effects experienced when taking the medication, fear of developing a serious complication caused by the medication, lack of understanding of the purpose of the medication, and financial limitations. The latter barrier can often be overcome by accessing the special programs available from the pharmaceutical companies that manufacture these medications, which are intended to help patients offset the costs of these expensive medications.

(See the Resources of Benefit section at the end of this book for more details.)

When a woman is initially diagnosed with breast cancer, she wants to do all that she can to rid herself of the disease and reduce her risk of recurrence. As more time goes by and the patient is past the period when the risk of recurrence is its highest (the first 2 years), she may begin weighing the pros and cons of taking medications that are causing her unpleasant side effects against the benefit of reducing her risk. Quality of life is a priority for these women—as it should be. As healthcare professionals, we need to help our patients find a sense of balance in reducing the risk of recurrence while maintaining an active, enjoyable lifestyle—with both parties working cooperatively, with our patients' understanding and involvement in this process.

Frequently Asked Questions

1. ***What are the primary side effects of hormonal therapy that concern women?***

   The precise side effects depend on the specific drug. More generally, hormonal therapy tends to produce menopausal symptoms such as hot flashes, vaginal dryness, lower libido, night sweats, sexual dysfunction, and mood swings. These symptoms can be sufficiently severe to truly diminish a woman's quality of life. It is important for the healthcare provider to provide medications or other resources that can help reduce these side effects.

2. ***What is the key issue to emphasize to patients who are taking hormonal therapy?***

   Providers must reinforce the importance of taking the medication as prescribed. Hormonal therapy drugs are taken for long periods and, therefore, are vulnerable to the same issues that arise with other medications prescribed for chronic diseases. In particular, noncompliance is an ongoing problem. The patient should be educated so that she understands the benefit she is receiving by taking the medication—namely, the reduction in her risk of recurrence of breast cancer; this message cannot be underemphasized.

3. ***What can be done about the side effect of potential bone loss caused by AIs? Is a woman's risk of osteoporosis (e.g., because of family history or previous bone density studies confirming osteopenia) reason to not prescribe or discontinue an AI?***

   It is increasingly common practice to prescribe a bisphosphonate for the patient to take with an AI, with the goal of preventing AI-related osteoporosis. Family history of osteoporosis or personal history of osteopenia has not been found to be a contraindication to taking AI as the hormonal therapy of choice.

4. ***Which issues related to birth control should be discussed with a patient who is taking hormonal therapy?***

   Even if her menstrual periods stop as a result of taking hormonal therapy (such as tamoxifen), the patient cannot assume that she is not ovulating. Therefore, birth control should be practiced by all sexually active, premenopausal women who are taking hormonal therapy. For women who were perimenopausal at the time they began their hormonal therapy, appropriate blood tests should be done to definitively determine their menopausal status before declaring that these patients are postmenopausal. Hormonal therapy carries a risk of birth defects if women become pregnant while taking one of these drugs, so the importance of practicing contraception should be emphasized.

REFERENCES

1. Miller NH. Compliance with treatment regimens in chronic asymptomatic diseases. *Am J Med.* 1997;102 (2A):43–49.
2. World Health Organization. *Adherence to long-term therapies: evidence for action.* Geneva, Switzerland: WHO Publications; 2003:211.
3. Osterberg L, Blaschke T. Adherence to medication. *N Engl J Med.* 2005;353:487–497.
4. National Cancer Institute. Tamoxifen: questions and answers.http://www.cancer.gov/cancertopics/factsheet/Therapy/tamoxifen. Accessed September 15, 2009.
5. Goss PE, Ingle JN, Martino S, et al. Efficacy of letrozole extended therapy according to estrogen receptor and progesterone receptor status of the primary tumor: National Cancer Institute of Canada Clinical Trials Group MA.17. *J Clin Oncol.* 2007;25(15):2006–2011.

6. Buzdar AV, Baum M, Cuzick J. Letrozole or tamoxifen in early breast cancer. *N Engl J Med.* 2006;354(14): 1528–1530; author reply 1528–1530.
7. Wardley AM. Emerging data on optimal adjuvant endocrine therapy: Breast International Group Trial 1–98/MA.17. *Clin Breast Cancer.* 2006;6(suppl 2): S45–S50.
8. Loprinzi C, Stearns V, Barton D. Centrally active nonhormonal hot flash therapies. *Am J Med.* 2005;118 (12B):118S–123S.
9. Kendall A, Dowestt M, Folkerd E, Smith I. Caution: vaginal estradiol appears to be contraindicated in post-menopausal women on adjuvant aromatase inhibitors. *Annals Oncol.* 2006;17(4):584–587.
10. Bender BG, Bender SE. Patient-identified barriers to treatment adherence: responses to interviews, focus groups, and questionnaires. *Immunol Allergy Clin North Am.* 2005;25:107–130.
11. Wirk B. The role of ovarian ablation in the management of breast cancer. *Breast J.* 2005;11(6):416–424.
12. Joant W, Pritchard KI, Sainsbury R, Klijn JG. Trends in endocrine therapy and chemotherapy for early-stage breast cancer: a focus on the postmenopausal patient. *J Cancer Res Clin Oncol* 2006;132(5):275–286.
13. Goldstein LJ. Controversies in adjuvant endocrine treatment of premenopausal women. *Clin Breast Cancer.* 2006;6(suppl 2):S36–S40.

FURTHER READING

Kalow W (Ed.). *Pharmacogenetics of drug metabolism.* New York: Pergamon Press; 1992.

Novartis Foundation. *From genome to therapy: integrating new technologies with drug development.* New York: John Wiley; 2000.

Wilkes GM. *Pocket guide to breast cancer drugs.* Sudbury, MA: Jones and Bartlett; 2005.

ACKNOWLEDGMENTS

The author would like to thank Dr. Vered Stearns, at Johns Hopkins, and Dr. James Rae at the University of Michigan, for their input to the pharmacogenetics section of this chapter.

CHAPTER 6

Algorithm for Women at High Risk

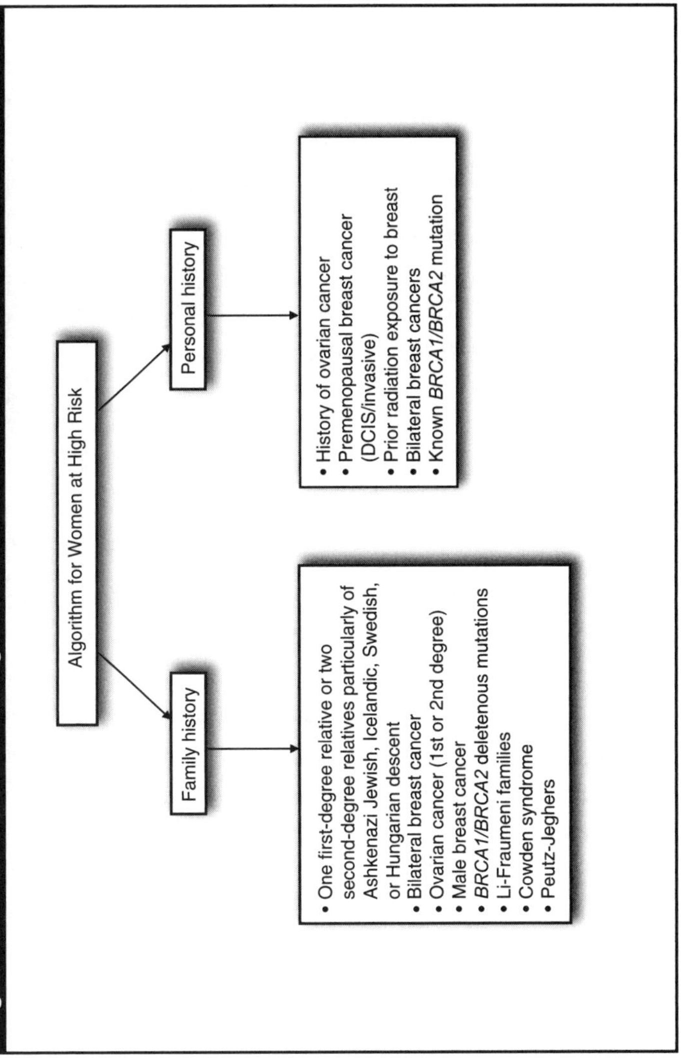

CHAPTER 6

A Practical Approach to Assessing High-Risk Women

Kala Visvanathan, MD, BS, FRACP, MHS
Lillie Shockney, RN, BS, MAS

What you need to know:

At the time your patient was diagnosed and underwent treatment for her breast cancer, she would have also undergone an assessment of her risk for carrying a gene that predisposed her to getting this disease. It is important to continue to ask her questions about her family history. Initially she may not have had any relatives with breast or ovarian cancer; however, 4 years later she may have had a sister or mother diagnosed. This medical history information is important to keep up to date; therefore, each time you see her, ask her to provide information associated with any relatives who have been diagnosed with cancer since you last saw her.

If you are considering referring a patient for assessment of breast cancer risk factors (which may include genetic testing), screening, and risk-reduction options owing to family or personal history, plan to provide the following medical information so that the doctor and genetic counselor seeing her can accurately do the assessment requested:

- Family history of breast cancer in first- or second-degree relatives
- Detailed gynecologic and breast surgical history, as well as radiological history
- Medical history including risk factors: age at first menstrual period, age at menopause, age at birth of first child, history of atypical hyperplasia, history of breast biopsies, race, knowledge of prior genetic testing in her family, personal history of cancers

Although 20% to 30% of women may have a family history of breast cancer, only 5% to 10% have a hereditary predisposition toward this disease.

Women who carry deleterious mutations in the BRCA1 or BRCA2 genes are counseled about preventive steps to take to reduce their risk of developing cancer. Their risk during the lifetime is 36% to 85%; more detailed risk estimates are available based on age. Women are currently recommended to undergo prophylactic oophorectomy if they are past childbearing age because of the limited specificity of current screening methods for ovarian cancer. In terms of breast cancer risk, options that are discussed with patients include increased screening (i.e., clinical breast examinations, mammograms, breast magnetic resonance imaging [MRI]), chemoprevention (tamoxifen), and prophylactic mastectomy. Data on the frequency and timing of MRI in such cases are currently being gathered. Based on existing data, however, it appears that prophylactic mastectomy can reduce the risk of breast cancer in high-risk women by 95%; prophylactic oophorectomy can reduce the risk by 80% to 90%.

Certain familial syndromes are associated with a higher risk of breast cancer, in addition to the deleterious mutations in the BRCA1 and BRCA2 genes. These conditions include Li-Fraumeni syndrome, Cowden syndrome, and Peutz-Jeghers syndrome.

There are specific clues that may be present in unaffected women, raising the possibility of them carrying a breast cancer gene. Table 6-1 lists these characteristics.

TABLE 6-1 Risk Factors for Breast Cancer

The following findings are important clues in women who are as yet unaffected by breast cancer, but who may have an inherited predisposition to breast cancer based on the family history of first- and second-degree relatives on either the maternal or paternal side, or both:
• More than one relative with early-onset breast cancer (younger than 50 years old)
• Bilateral breast cancer
• Male breast cancer
• Ovarian cancer at any age
• Breast and ovarian cancer in the same individual; bilateral breast cancer
• One relative with breast and/or ovarian cancer if the individual has any of the following ethnic backgrounds in whom founder mutations have been identified: Ashkenazi Jewish, Icelandic, Swedish, Hungarian

continues

TABLE 6-1 Risk Factors for Breast Cancer (*continued*)

• Family member with a known genetic mutation in a breast cancer susceptibility gene • History of multiple family members with pancreatic cancer, melanoma, prostate cancer, or gastric cancer • Cancer clusters of the following (not every cancer may be seen in the pedigree): ∘ Early-onset breast cancer, osteosarcoma, leukemia, brain tumors, adrenocortical malignancies, endometrial cancer (Li-Fraumeni syndrome) ∘ Early-onset breast cancer, nonmedullary thyroid cancer/ benign thyroid follicular adenoma or multinodular goiter; multiple hamartomatous lesions in skin (often at age 20 years), intestine, oral mucosa, or breast; prior history of benign breast disease (Cowden syndrome) ∘ Early-onset breast cancer; hamartomous polyps in gastrointestinal tract; melanin deposits in buccal mucosa, lips, fingers, and toes (Peutz-Jeghers syndrome)

What your patient needs to know:

Your patient needs to stay informed by her family members regarding others who may have been also diagnosed with cancers after she completed her treatment. This information needs to be conveyed to you to keep your medical records on her up to date in assessing her for the potential of carrying a breast cancer gene.

Your patient does not have control over her heredity and genetic makeup but she does have control over how she addresses her high-risk status.

Many women assume if they have a relative anywhere in their family tree with breast cancer, they are destined to get breast cancer. In fact, most women with a family history will not get this disease. Those at higher risk often have a family history that includes a first-degree relative or at least two second-degree relatives who were diagnosed at a relatively young age with breast cancer.

Genetic counseling and testing is available for two specific tumor-suppressor genes—BRCA1 and BRCA2. Other, less penetrant genes are likely to be identified in the future as factors in breast cancer development. Thus, if a woman's family history fits a specific pattern or she has developed breast cancer at an early age or has a history of ovarian cancer, she should be referred to a high-risk breast clinic for consideration of genetic testing. Where possible, genetic testing is undertaken on the person who is affected by breast cancer; if her test for the mutation is positive, then other healthy family members may undergo testing.

Women need genetic counseling and discussion of their risk before they embark on genetic testing. Although the test itself is simply a blood test, the ramifications of the results of the test need careful discussion before those results become known. For example, if testing would not change the patient's current management or be helpful for family members, then she might decide to postpone the test.

Certain syndromes put some women at higher risk for hereditary breast cancer. Having hereditary breast cancer may increase the risk of other types of cancers, such as ovarian cancer.

INTRODUCTION

This chapter is intended as a review of current clinical approaches used to identify healthy women at high risk for breast cancer and breast cancer survivors with family history to assist healthcare providers in giving risk-appropriate screening and management recommendations. It is increasingly common for a nurse practitioner to be following a breast cancer survivor as well as "adopt" other family members for breast health screening. Knowledge of a woman's breast cancer risk can be used to guide both screening and risk-reduction strategies. Such information can also decrease anxiety, particularly in young women with risk factors such as family history, as their perceived risk of developing breast cancer is often much higher than their actual risk. The overall goal of breast cancer risk assessment is twofold: (1) to target high-risk groups with more aggressive screening and risk-reduction strategies so as to increase their overall survival, and (2) to minimize overtreatment and its associated complications in low-risk groups.

At any age a woman can be classified as being at general population risk, at increased risk, or at high risk for breast cancer. The following medical, surgical, and family history information is needed to determine which risk group a woman fits into:

- Family history of cancer in first- and second-degree relatives on both the maternal and paternal sides
- Detailed gynecological and breast surgical history
- Medical history, including known breast cancer risk factors such as age at menarche, parity, age at

birth of first child, age at menopause (if occurred), history of previous breast biopsies, history of atypical hyperplasia, and race (in particular, whether there is any Ashkenazi Jewish heritage)

- Knowledge of any prior genetic testing in the family
- Information on any personal history of cancer

In practice, patients often may not remember or be able to provide this information immediately if asked at a clinic visit, particularly their family history. Therefore, requesting this information prior to the patient's appointment can be extremely helpful and efficient, and it can result in a more comprehensive and accurate assessment. It is also very important to ask the patient at least annually if there are any additional family members who have been diagnosed with cancer since you last saw her for a clinic visit. Her family profile when you first met her was not significant for depicting a possible genetic pattern but with more relatives diagnosed, it might be.

It is reasonable to perform a baseline risk assessment when a woman is between the ages of 18 and 20 years to determine whether she has a strong family history of breast cancer or possible hereditary syndrome that might affect her breast cancer risk. Early identification of these women with a hereditary predisposition toward breast cancer is important, as they need to be more closely monitored with intense surveillance throughout their lifetime and may benefit from genetic testing and targeted risk-reduction strategies in their 20s. A woman's breast cancer risk should be regularly reevaluated over her lifetime, because many of the known risk factors (including family history and age) will change over time and with the woman's experiences.

IDENTIFICATION OF WOMEN AT HIGH RISK FOR BREAST CANCER

Family history of breast cancer is an important risk factor on its own. A woman with a first-degree relative with breast cancer has a two- to threefold increased risk of developing breast cancer as compared to women with no such family history. This risk increases to fourfold if there is more than one first-degree relative with breast cancer. Although 20% to 30% of women report having at least one relative with breast cancer, only 5% to 10% have what is known as a hereditary predisposition, which places them at high risk for breast cancer (Table 6-2). For women with any one of these rare inherited syndromes, the risk of developing breast cancer in their lifetime ranges from 22% to 85%. Age-specific estimates of this risk play an important role when discussing management options. These women are

TABLE 6-2 Inherited Syndromes Associated with a High Risk of Early-Onset Breast Cancer

Familial Syndrome	Gene Involved	Other Associated Conditions
Breast/ovarian	BRCA1/BRCA2	Ovarian, pancreas, prostate, melanoma, and male breast cancers
Li-Fraumeni syndrome	p53	Bone or soft-tissue sarcoma, leukemia, brain tumors, and adrenocortical malignancies, childhood cancers, adenocarcinoma
Cowden syndrome	PTEN	Mucocutaneous lesions of the face and oral mucosa,

continues

TABLE 6-2 Inherited Syndromes Associated with a High Risk of Early-Onset Breast Cancer (*continued*)

Familial Syndrome	Gene Involved	Other Associated Conditions
		cerebellar tumors, benign and malignant (nonmedullary) thyroid cancer, endometrial cancer, macrocephaly, mental retardation, multiple hamartomas of the gastrointestinal tract, uterine fibromas, benign breast lesions, lipomas
Peutz-Jeghers syndrome	STK11	Hamartomous polyps in gastrointestinal tract; freckles in buccal mucosa, lips, fingers, and toes; thyroid cancer; ovarian cancer including sex cord tumors

also at risk for other cancers and related benign conditions. The chance that they develop at least one type of cancer in their lifetime is close to 90%.

BRCA GENES

The majority of known hereditary breast cancers are due to deleterious mutations in the BRCA1 and BRCA2 genes. These tumor suppressor genes are involved in DNA repair. The BRCA1 gene is located on chromosome 17, and the BRCA2 gene is found on chromosome 13. An individual has two copies of each gene, one from each parent. Deleterious mutations in each gene are inherited in an autosomal dominant manner. Mutations in BRCA1 are thought to explain 90% of breast and ovarian cancers observed in families and 45% of multiple breast cancer cases.

In the general population, the prevalence of BRCA mutations is rare, occurring in 0.1% of women. Specific familial mutations in these genes are more common in certain populations, such as Ashkenazi Jewish women. The lifetime risk of breast cancer among women who are mutation carriers has been estimated to be between 36% and 85%, according to reported studies from different study populations. The lifetime risk of ovarian cancer is between 16% and 60% in the same population. Mutation carriers also have an increased risk of second breast cancers. Men with deleterious mutations in these two genes are also at increased risk for male breast cancer and prostate cancer, albeit to a lesser degree. Melanoma and pancreatic cancers in some families have also been linked to these mutations.

Genetic testing for mutations in these two genes is available. Screening guidelines have been developed for BRCA mutation carriers based on the opinions of expert groups. Young women in families in which there is a known mutation should be encouraged to perform breast self-examinations from the age 18 years onward; from age 25 years or at the point when they are 10 years younger than the age of the individual in the family when first diagnosed with the breast cancer, they should begin having clinical breast exams between two and four times a year and mammograms and MRIs annually. The optimal frequency and duration of both mammography and MRI screening in high-risk women is not known. There is some concern about long-term radiation exposure with mammography in this group; this issue needs to be further elucidated.

Higher sensitivities in detecting breast cancer have been reported with MRI compared to mammogram but lower specificities. Therefore, MRI is currently being used as a screening tool only in high-risk women. It is also not known whether routine MRI screening in BRCA mutation carriers is associated with increased survival.

The option of prophylactic mastectomy with or without reconstruction is also discussed as a potential risk-reduction strategy for BRCA mutation carriers. On the basis of results of retrospective and prospective studies, prophylactic mastectomy appears to decrease the risk of developing breast cancer by approximately 90% in women at high risk. Long-term prospective studies are ongoing.

In practice, more women tend to choose screening over bilateral prophylactic mastectomy. Unilateral prophylactic mastectomy is also an option for BRCA mutation carriers diagnosed with breast cancer. There may also be a role for chemoprevention with tamoxifen, a selective estrogen-receptor modulator (SERM), in both premenopausal and postmenopausal BRCA mutation carriers. Only a few small studies have evaluated the benefit of tamoxifen as a chemopreventive agent specifically in BRCA mutation carriers. These studies have been inconclusive owing to limited sizes. It is believed that BRCA2 mutation carriers may receive a greater benefit from tamoxifen than BRCA1 mutation carriers do, as the former are more likely to develop estrogen receptor-positive tumors, which are known to be prevented by tamoxifen. In the clinical setting, it is important to present both the risks and the benefits of tamoxifen when discussing it as an option for breast cancer risk reduction in at-risk women. As yet, there are no data on the chemopreventive benefits offered by either raloxifene (another SERM) or aromatase inhibitors (AIs) in postmenopausal BRCA mutation carriers.

Given the lack of efficacy of screening approaches for ovarian cancer (in particular, the shortcomings of serum CA125 levels and transvaginal ultrasound for this purpose), it is currently recommended that BRCA mutation carriers undergo prophylactic bilateral salpingo-oophorectomy (BSO) after they have completed childbearing and are older than 35 years of age. The fallopian tubes should be removed in addition to the ovaries because of the increased risk of fallopian tube carcinoma in BRCA mutation carriers. Whether the uterus should be removed, given that a small part of the fallopian tube resides there, is still controversial. Ongoing prospective studies may help answer this question. We suggest that the surgery be done by a trained gynecologist/oncologist or with one present who could carry out the surgery if required, as early-stage ovarian cancer has been detected in a small percentage of these cases. In BRCA mutation carriers, prophylactic BSO has been associated with as much as a 50% decrease in breast cancer in premenopausal patients.

Another controversial issue is whether premenopausal women should receive hormone replacement therapy (HRT) postoophorectomy and, if so, for how long. A number of clinics use short-term hormonal therapy only in women with severe vasomotor symptoms while others give low-dose hormone therapy until the average age of menopause. Women with a history of melanoma or fair skin should undergo annual skin examination. Men with BRCA mutations should have annual breast exams and prostate-specific antigen (PSA) levels measured at 40 years of age.

LI-FRAUMENI SYNDROME

The Li-Fraumeni syndrome is a rare autosomal dominant condition in which members of a family have early-onset breast cancer, osteosarcoma, leukemia, brain tumors, and adrenocortical malignancies. In Li-Fraumeni families, the reported incidence of early-onset breast cancer is as high as 22%, and women are often susceptible to having multiple breast cancers in addition to other cancers. In approximately 50% to 77% of cases, a mutation in the p53 gene has been detected. The p53 gene is located on chromosome 17 and is responsible for a number of cellular functions including cell growth. Testing for a mutation in the p53 gene can be undertaken. Breast cancer screening guidelines for p53 mutation carriers are similar to those for BRCA mutation carriers. Prophylactic mastectomies are also an option. It is suggested that women in Li-Fraumeni families undergo comprehensive annual physical examinations given their risk of other cancers.

COWDEN SYNDROME

Cowden syndrome is another rare autosomal dominant syndrome characterized by a cluster of benign and malignant conditions: mucocutaneous lesions on the face and oral mucosa; early-onset breast cancer; benign and malignant (nonmedullary) thyroid cancer; macrocephaly; cerebellar tumors; endometrial cancer; mental retardation; hamartomas of the gastrointestinal tract; benign breast lesions; lipomas; renal carcinoma; and uterine fibroids.

Cowden syndrome is the result of a deleterious mutation in the PTEN (phosphatase and tensin homolog) tumor suppressor gene. Testing for mutations in the PTEN gene is available.

In PTEN mutation carriers, skin lesions often present first, at an early age. Early-onset breast cancer develops in 25% to 50% of female carriers. Women can present with bilateral breast cancer. A prior history of benign breast disease is also common.

Breast cancer screening recommendations for PTEN mutation carriers are the same as those for BRCA mutation carriers. Prophylactic mastectomy is also a risk-reduction option. In premenopausal women, endometrial biopsies are recommended every 5 years beginning between the ages of 35 and 40 years and continuing until menopause; thereafter, annual ultrasounds should be performed. In addition, an annual physical examination including urinalysis, annual thyroid ultrasound, and skin examination is recommended.

PEUTZ-JEGHERS SYNDROME

Peutz-Jeghers syndrome is a rare autosomal dominant condition characterized by freckles in infancy that may fade with age and hamartomatous polyps in the gastrointestinal tract. It is also associated with a 50% risk of developing breast cancer, in addition to an increased risk of colon, pancreas, stomach, and ovarian cancers (including sex cord tumors). In 50% of cases, germline mutations in STK11 at chromosome 19 (also known as LKB1) are identified. Genetic testing for this syndrome is available.

Women with Peutz-Jeghers are recommended to undergo clinical breast examinations beginning at age 20 and mammograms at age 40. Annual Pap smears and transvaginal ultrasound should begin when women are teenagers. In addition, an annual comprehensive physical examination is recommended. Men with Peutz-Jeghers syndrome should have annual testicular examinations starting at age 20.

WOMEN WITHOUT A FAMILY HISTORY OF BREAST CANCER

The following criteria are used to identify women at increased risk for breast cancer who do not have a strong family history:

- Women 35 years or older with a 5-year breast cancer risk of 1.66% or greater (derived using the National Cancer Institute Breast Cancer Risk Assessment Model; www.cancer.gov/bcrisktool)
- Women with a prior diagnosis of lobular carcinoma in situ (LCIS) or atypical hyperplasia
- Women with a prior history of radiation exposure

With the exception of women who have a prior history of thoracic radiation, recommended screening strategies in women at increased risk are similar to those used for the general population. In the United States, that means clinical breast examinations every 1 to 3 years between the ages of 20 and 40, followed by the addition of mammograms every 1 to 2 years between ages 40 and 50 and annually thereafter (see Agency for Healthcare Research and Quality for additional information about screening guidelines: http://www.ahrq.gov/clinic/uspstf/uspsbrca.htm). Some healthcare providers advise semiannual clinical breast examinations.

Women who have a history of thoracic radiation are currently recommended to undergo annual clinical breast examinations before the age of 25, and breast self-examinations with annual mammograms beginning 10 years after the completion of radiation or at age 40, whichever comes first. Although data suggest that a woman's breast cancer risk varies based on her current age, radiation dose, and use of chemotherapy, these findings have not yet been translated into clinical practice. These women need to be followed closely, which can also be done by a high-risk breast clinic. As yet, no study has evaluated the benefit of annual MRI in this population.

In addition to screening, women 35 years or older with a 5-year breast cancer risk of 1.66% or greater (derived using the NCI Breast Cancer Risk Assessment Model) or with a history of LCIS or atypical hyperplasia may benefit from chemopreventive strategies such as tamoxifen (in premenopausal and postmenopausal women) or raloxifene (in postmenopausal women). Patients can also be referred to a high-risk breast clinic for discussion of the risks and benefits of these chemopreventive strategies.

It is appropriate to refer women diagnosed with early-onset breast cancer (younger than 50 years) without a family history and women with bilateral breast cancers, second breast cancers, and ovarian cancer to a high-risk breast clinic for risk assessment, possible genetic testing, and management recommendations.

GUIDELINES FOR ASSESSMENT AND TREATMENT OF HIGH-RISK WOMEN

Expert guidelines from groups such as the U.S. Preventive Services Task Force and the National Comprehensive Cancer Network (NCCN) have been developed to assist physicians and other healthcare providers in identifying women who, based on family history of cancer, may have an inherited breast cancer predisposition.

The criteria listed in Table 6-1 can be used to identify women who should be referred to a high-risk breast clinic for one or more of the hereditary breast cancer syndromes. Information on high-risk breast clinics is available on the Web sites of most National Cancer Institute (NCI)–designated Comprehensive Cancer Centers and many university-affiliated breast centers. These facilities can provide a more detailed risk assessment as well as genetic counseling and testing, breast examination and tailored screening, and risk-reduction strategies for women who are at increased risk of breast and ovarian cancers. Their staffs usually include both genetic counselors and medical oncologists/internists. When genetic testing is an option, testing of a family member affected with cancer is preferred; unaffected members would then be tested only if a mutation was found. Patients and/or family members who come to these clinics also often have the opportunity to be involved with ongoing research studies. The following Web sites may also be helpful in locating a high-risk breast clinic:

- http://www.cancer.gov/cancercenters/centerslist.html
- http://www.facingourrisk.org/finding_health_care/finding_specialists.html#clinics

- http://www.cancer.gov/search/results_geneticsservices.aspx

Women with a strong family history (based on the criteria outlined in Table 6-1) but no identified genetic mutation are usually managed similarly to BRCA mutation carriers. For the remaining women with a family history, annual clinical breast examination and mammogram screening are usually recommended to begin 10 years before the first case of breast cancer was diagnosed in the family, except if the diagnosis of breast cancer occurred while the family member was in her early 20s. MRI is currently not recommended for these women.

Frequently Asked Questions

1. ***Once a patient is confirmed to have a deleterious BRCA1 or BRCA2 mutation, how urgent is it for her to take action if she is considering prophylactic surgery?***

   Under normal circumstances, other than increasing intensity of breast and ovarian surveillance, it is not urgent for her to take action. In fact, a woman is advised to take the time to gather opinions and discuss options with treating physicians and family members when considering all risk-reduction options. The only scenario that requires immediate action is when a patient who has breast cancer and is found to be positive for a BRCA mutation is considering bilateral mastectomies and reconstruction. This is because specific types of breast reconstruction, such as deep inferior epigastric perforator (DIEP) flaps, can be done only once. If this is the case, the patient should discuss this issue with her breast and plastic surgeon and be referred to a high-risk breast clinic as soon as possible, as it can take between 4 and 6 weeks to get genetic test results back pending insurance authorization.

2. ***How young is it reasonable to test a patient for mutations in the BRCA1 and BRCA2 genes?***

We usually recommend delaying testing until at least the mid-20s, when it may affect the choice of screening strategies. In making this decision, we also take into consideration the maturity, emotional state, and wishes of the individual. We do recommend that women be seen at a high-risk breast clinic to discuss their risk and guide screening strategies, and also so that they can be informed of ongoing changes in practice as the field evolves. This can be done earlier if they are aware of their family's history of breast cancer.

At present we recommend that young women in families of known BRCA mutation carriers, who have not been tested themselves, perform monthly breast self-examinations from age 18 onward and undergo annual clinical breast examinations as part of their annual physical examinations. In addition, we recommend that at age 25, women in this group begin semiannual clinical breast examinations, annual mammograms, and MRIs. The starting age may be lowered if there is a very early onset of breast cancer in the family.

3. ***Is BRCA genetic testing covered by insurance?***

Insurance reimbursement may vary from country to country and from place to place. In the United States, most insurance companies cover at least 80% of the cost of genetic testing. Each insurance company has its own set of criteria. If testing is believed to be clinically required, a letter of medical necessity can be sent to the insurance company.

4. ***Does being BRCA positive affect a patient's health insurance or life insurance?***

In the United States, the Health Insurance Portability and Accounting Act of 1996 (HIPAA) prevents group health coverage from either excluding individuals or increasing their premiums as a result of genetic testing results. However, the same rule does not apply to individual insurance coverage. In addition, HIPAA does not prevent health insurance companies from asking about prior genetic testing.

A number of states developed laws some time ago prohibiting group health plans from discriminating on the basis of genetic testing results; some states also have legislation preventing employers from discriminating on the basis of genetic testing results. Though it took 13 years to get a federal law passed, we now have the GINA law—the Genetic

Information Nondiscrimination Act. This law will ensure that anyone who gets genetic tests will be protected from having that information shared with health insurers or employers.

The law will: (a) prohibit the use of genetic information to deny employment or insurance coverage; (b) ensure that genetic test results are kept private; and (c) prevent an insurer from basing eligibility or premiums on genetic information.

To date, it seems that genetic discrimination has not become a problem. Updated information on state-based cancer legislation can be obtained from the National Cancer Institute (www.scid-nci.net).

5. ***How long do BRCA mutation carriers have to be screened?***

Testing should occur intermittently throughout the patient's life. These patients should be connected to a high-risk breast clinic so that if imaging modalities or chemoprevention approaches change, they will be aware of this fact.

FURTHER READING

Claus EB, Risch N, Thompson WD. Autosomal dominant inheritance of early-onset breast cancer: implications for risk prediction. *Cancer.* 1994;73:643–651.

Fisher B, Constantino JP, Wickerham DL, et al. Tamoxifen for prevention of breast cancer: report of the National Surgical Adjuvant Breast and Bowel Project P-1 Study. *J Natl Cancer Inst.* 1993;90:1371–1388.

Gail MH, Brinton LA, Byar DP, et al. Projecting individualized probabilities of developing breast cancer for white females who are being examined annually. *J Natl Cancer Inst.* 1989;81:1879–1886.

WEB SITES

- http://www.ahrq.gov/clinic/uspstf/uspsbrca.htm
- http://www.cancer.gov/bcrisktool/
- http://www.cancer.org/docroot/home/index.asp
- http://www.cancer.gov/search/results_geneticsservices.aspx
- http://www.facingourrisk.org/finding_health_care/finding_specialists.html#clinics
- http://www.scid-nci.net

CHAPTER 7

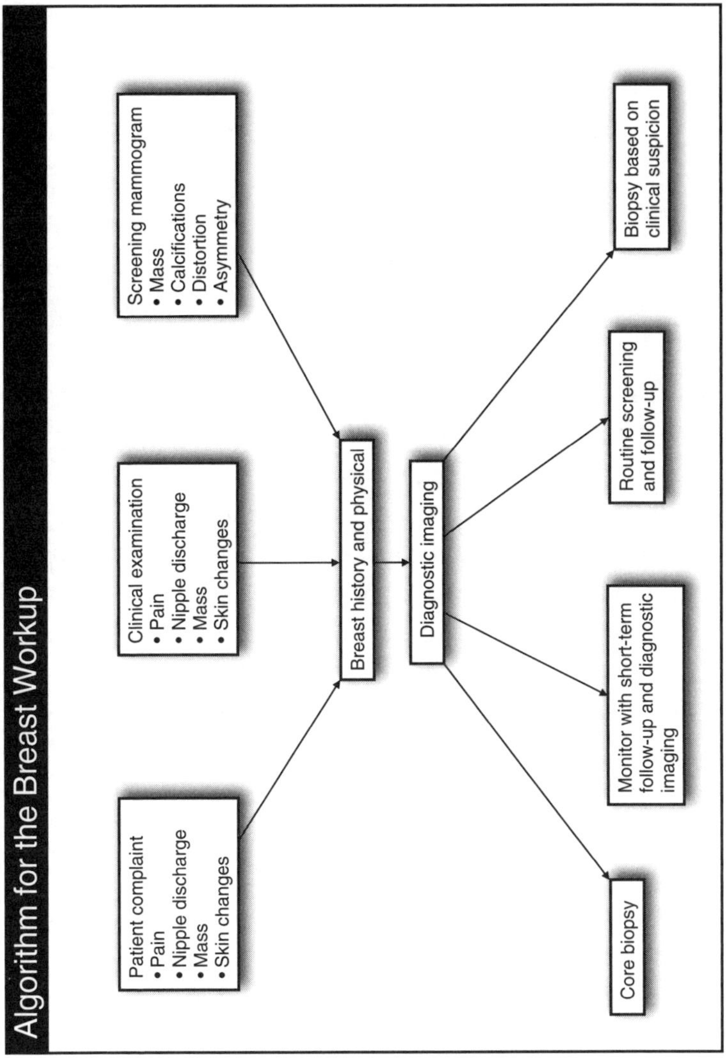

Algorithm for the Breast Workup
Patient complaint
• Pain
• Nipple discharge
• Mass
• Skin changes
Clinical examination
• Pain
• Nipple discharge
• Mass
• Skin changes
Screening mammogram
• Mass
• Calcifications
• Distortion
• Asymmetry
Breast history and physical
Diagnostic imaging
Core biopsy
Monitor with short-term follow-up and diagnostic imaging
Routine screening and follow-up
Biopsy based on clinical suspicion

CHAPTER 7

Benign Breast Disease

Theodore N. Tsangaris, MD

What you need to know:

Breast cancer survivors are not immune to developing or already having benign breast conditions. In some cases, this patient population may have more breast abnormalities on imaging studies and clinical breast exams due simply to the fact that they have already been diagnosed and treated for breast cancer.

It should be expected that breast cancer survivors will worry if they find an abnormality on breast self-exam and may assume that it is the cancer having recurred.

Every breast problem should be approached in a consistent way. The three basic elements include history, physical examination, and diagnostic imaging.

A diagnostic mammogram should be ordered for any breast problem. This type of imaging study can and should be obtained even before the patient sees a breast surgeon. The healthcare provider should provide as much pertinent information as possible to aid the mammographer in the workup.

All breast problems should be approached with a high index of suspicion and with the goal of ruling out breast cancer.

What your patient needs to know:

Most problems of the breast are benign. However, patients should be encouraged to bring any issues to the attention of their healthcare provider. Usually breast cancer survivors are very good about bringing to their provider's attention the development of a new symptom, out of fear it is recurrence of the disease.

Breast self-examination is important in providing information about stability in a clinical finding. It may also aid the clinician and the mammographer in their workup.

Patients should be reassured about the safety and efficacy of the core biopsy as the procedure of choice when a biopsy is necessary.

INTRODUCTION

The specific entity of benign breast disease does not exist. Rather, benign breast disease is a collection of symptoms with or without corresponding pathological findings. These symptoms are relatively unimportant as pathologic findings and are often collectively termed "fibrocystic disease."[1]

There are few effective treatments for these symptoms or pathologic findings. Surgery for this group of entities is usually not indicated but is almost always used as a diagnostic tool. Frankly, your patient will be interested in just two diagnoses of the breast when faced with a problem: cancer and "not cancer" (i.e., benign disease). Specifics and treatment of benign disease are usually not important to the patient once she hears "not cancer." Therefore, it is most important for the clinician to approach all symptoms or findings in the breast with the ultimate goal of making the diagnosis of cancer or "not cancer." This chapter describes the presenting symptoms of benign breast disease and explains how to make the diagnosis of cancer or "not cancer" (benign).

GENERAL APPROACH TO THE BREAST PROBLEM

There are three ways a breast problem will present itself to the clinician. First are the symptoms or findings identified by the patient during her breast self-examination (BSE). BSE is often maligned as a screening tool, but it is still a common way that a woman identifies a breast cancer. In addition, the familiarity of the state of her breast gained from routine BSE that a woman brings to an encounter with her physician or mammographer is invaluable. Second, a problem may present itself during a clinical breast examination performed by the patient's healthcare provider. Third, findings may present during breast imaging, usually during a screening mammogram.

Regardless of how the issue is identified, the same principles apply. A good history is appropriate in all situations. Attention to personal breast history, family breast history, and gynecologic history are the mainstays of the pertinent information (although most women with breast cancer have no known risk factors). A skilled breast examination follows the history. Consistency in technique is more important than the mechanics of this examination. Usually the breast examination begins on the contralateral breast so that a "normal breast" can be established for direct comparison to the breast with the problem. The breast tissue technically extends from the clavicle superiorly, to just below the inframammary fold inferiorly. It extends from the lateral edge of the sternum medially and to the posterior axillary line or latissimus muscle laterally. A complete breast examination includes both breasts as well as the axillary nodes and the supraclavicular nodes.

The workup of a breast problem always includes breast imaging. No matter what the issue under investigation, failure to obtain appropriate breast imaging would be considered a deviation from the standard of care. The primary healthcare provider overseeing her survivorship care should feel comfortable in ordering a diagnostic breast-imaging study prior to the patient seeing a breast surgeon. Not only is this step appropriate, but it will facilitate the surgeon's workup should his or her services be needed.

What constitutes appropriate imaging is another story. Therefore, a word about obtaining a diagnostic mammogram is appropriate here. Designating the study as a "diagnostic" workup in the request is the first and most important component. Inherent in the word *diagnostic* is the implication that a qualified breast imager will oversee the process from beginning to end. Additional views, ultrasounds, or other imaging modalities such as magnetic resonance imaging (MRI) will be employed under the watchful eye of the breast imager. This also gives him or her permission to continue the workup to its conclusion—even to perform a biopsy if needed.

Communication with a breast imager by providing the relevant history and clinical information is paramount in facilitating the correct imaging workup. Thus an accurate description of the symptoms or findings on the requisition form is the second most important component of the imaging study. It is the responsibility of the ordering healthcare provider to be clear about the purpose of the study and to provide pertinent history and clinical findings to aid the breast imager in his or her task. The most common way to relay the location of a clinical finding is by using the coordinates of the clock. Of course, if all else fails, a simple crude drawing can be very effective.

The mammographer should take the workup to its conclusion by reaching one of the following end points:

- The mammographer may perform a core biopsy.
- The mammographer may make a recommendation for excisional biopsy.
- The mammographer may recommend a follow-up study.
- The mammographer may recommend continued regular screening.

Mammography is not infallible; it may miss as many as 15% of cancers for reasons related to the patient's age and breast density. Therefore, it is up to the clinician to pursue clinical findings of concern, even in the face of normal imaging studies. If biopsy is recommended, then core biopsy is preferred. Suffice it to say that core biopsy is minimally invasive, is highly accurate, and preserves breast integrity should subsequent procedures be necessary.

Excisional biopsy is reserved for instances in which core biopsy cannot be performed or for discordance between core biopsy results and clinical impression. The algorithm at the beginning of this chapter illustrates the basic approach to a breast problem.[2-4]

BREAST PAIN

Breast pain may be the most common complaint a woman will associate with her breast. Unfortunately, it is often the most difficult and frustrating to diagnose and treat. Although pain is not the usual presenting sign of cancer, when cancer is the cause of breast pain it is usually of an advanced stage. Reassurance is very important and often is the most important part of treatment. Breast pain should be taken seriously, however, and the usual workup initially outlined in this chapter should ensue. First, a thorough history and clinical breast examination should be done. Often the culprit is identified in the history. Regardless of the findings, a diagnostic mammogram should be obtained.[5]

Causes of breast pain include the influence of endogenous hormones (e.g., the menstrual cycle) or exogenous hormones (oral contraceptives and hormone replacement therapy). Stimulation of the breast from well-known culprits such as caffeine, chocolate, and soft drinks is not unusual. Again, the therapeutic value of reassurance cannot be overstated. Removing the offending cause, if one is identified, can bring about relief. Heat, vitamin E, evening primrose oil, and nonsteroidal anti-inflammatory drugs (NSAIDs) are all reasonable options, but hearing the words *not cancer* may be the most effective medicine.[6]

Assuming that the clinical examination and mammographic workup are negative, follow-up examinations and imaging are warranted at prescribed intervals or sooner should there be any change in the patient's clinical signs or symptoms. Surgery for pain of unknown etiology is strongly discouraged. Rarely does the patient obtain pain relief after the surgery, and most often the clinical picture is complicated by the addition of postsurgical pain and changes.

Table 7-1 summarizes the common causes, diagnosis, and treatment of breast pain.

TABLE 7-1 Breast Pain: A Summary

Common Causes
Menstrual cycle
Exogenous hormones
Coffee or tea
Chocolate
Soft drinks or other caffeine sources
Mass or cyst
Cancer (rare, and usually advanced at the point of causing pain)
Diagnosis
History
Physical examination
Mammogram/ultrasound
Biopsy as needed
Treatment
Reassurance
Vitamin E, evening primrose oil, nonsteroidal anti-inflammatory drugs, heat
Remove offending cause
Cyst aspiration
Excision of mass

NIPPLE DISCHARGE

Contrary to popular belief, nipple discharge is common and usually benign. Of all the causes of nipple discharge, breast cancer is the least common. The anxiety of patients and healthcare providers increases when the nature of the discharge is crystal clear and sticky, or bloody. Even in these scenarios, however, cancer is the least common cause of bloody nipple discharge; the two most common causes are duct ectasia and intraductal papilloma.

The usual thorough history and physical examination are necessary in patients who experience nipple discharge. In addition to identifying the discharge, the clinical examination should seek other findings such as a mass or a trigger point. A trigger point is the particular area of the breast that, upon palpation or manipulation, reproduces the discharge. A mass may or may not be associated with the trigger point.

A diagnostic mammogram is also a necessary component of the workup. A duct-o-gram may be helpful in these situations.[6] The finding of an abnormality on either mammogram or ultrasound is important. For benign nipple discharge (bilateral, nonbloody, multiple ducts), reassurance is appropriate with follow-up. Nipple discharge of concern (unilateral, single duct, bloody, or any discharge associated with clinical or mammographic abnormality) should be treated with a nipple duct exploration and/or biopsy of the associated clinical or mammographic abnormality.[7]

Table 7-2 summarizes the common causes, diagnosis, and treatment of nipple discharge.

TABLE 7-2 Nipple Discharge: A Summary

Common Causes
Benign and physiologic
Duct ectasia
Intraductal papilloma
Cancer
Diagnosis
History
Clinical examination (mass, trigger point)
Mammogram/ultrasound and duct-o-gram (mass, calcifications, distortion, filling defect)
Treatment
Observation
Biopsy as needed
Nipple duct exploration

NIPPLE CHANGES

Nipple changes such as itching, scaling, change in color, and erosion could be early signs of breast cancer and warrant a complete breast workup. Nipple changes, even in the face of a normal breast examination or mammogram, may require a biopsy to diagnose occult breast cancer.

Table 7-3 summarizes the common causes, diagnosis, and treatment of nipple changes.

RASHES AND OTHER SKIN CHANGES

The breast is covered by skin and, therefore, skin rashes are possible. These conditions should not be neglected—a heightened level of suspicion should prevail. A careful history, examination, and mammogram are mandatory.

TABLE 7-3 Nipple Changes: A Summary

Common Causes
Benign skin lesions
Trauma
Early sign of breast cancer
Diagnosis
History
Physical examination
Mammogram/ultrasound
Biopsy of nipple
Treatment
Treat the underlying cause

After a reasonable period of observation and consultation by a dermatologist, if needed, the persistence of the problem should initiate a workup that includes a punch biopsy to determine if these symptoms are a sign of inflammatory breast cancer. Patients who had locally advanced disease and/or previous history of inflammatory breast cancer should have a skin punch biopsy done early on when symptoms are noted.

It is never considered normal to have a breast infection. All breast infections have an underlying cause and should be treated with a high index of suspicion. In women of childbearing age, women who are pregnant, and nursing mothers, physiologic bases for the infection are reasonable considerations. In all other women, and particularly in perimenopausal and postmenopausal women, a breast infection should be considered breast cancer until proven otherwise.

A short course of antibiotics is reasonable provided that a clinical examination and diagnostic mammogram are performed immediately. Inflammatory breast cancer is often confused with a benign breast infection. A delay in recognizing the true etiology of the skin changes caused from this virulent form of breast cancer can be catastrophic.

Dimpling, skin retraction, changes in color, and swelling should initiate the workup cascade for the breast previously mentioned in this chapter.

Table 7-4 summarizes the common causes, diagnosis, and treatment of rashes and other skin changes.

BREAST MASSES

Masses may present to the patient during BSE, the nurse during clinical examination, or the radiologist during

TABLE 7-4 Rashes and Other Skin Changes: A Summary

Common Causes
Infection in nursing women and women of childbearing age
Generalized skin conditions
Cancer (maintain a high index of suspicion)
Diagnosis
History
Physical examination
Mammogram/ultrasound
Treatment
Short course of antibiotics or treatment by a dermatologist
Low threshold for further workup and biopsy

breast imaging. Regardless of their presentation, all dominant or isolated breast masses require evaluation, although not all masses need to be surgically removed. Masses that are suspicious in character or that are changing require biopsy. If a mass is clinically apparent, then breast imaging is warranted; if it is mammographically detected, then a clinical examination is appropriate.

Masses may generally be divided into cystic (fluid filled), solid (no fluid), or complex cyst (solid and cystic). A cyst should be aspirated if it is painful, enlarging, or changing, or if the diagnosis of a simple cyst is in question. Most dominant or isolated solid masses should be biopsied with either a core biopsy or fine-needle aspiration (FNA). Excisional biopsies should be reserved for equivocal core biopsies or lesions not amenable to FNA or core biopsy. Incisional biopsies should almost never be performed.

Keep in mind that initially postsurgery as well as post-radiation a patient may develop various changes to her breast tissue that can feel like an abnormality when comparing it to a presurgical or preradiation therapy clinical breast exam. Changes are to be expected for several months following local treatment of this nature.

A mass may be followed clinically and/or with imaging without surgical intervention if it has benign features, has shown stability over time, or has benign cytology on FNA or core biopsy.

Table 7-5 summarizes the common causes, diagnosis, and treatment of breast masses.

TABLE 7-5 Breast Rashes: A Summary

Common Causes
Benign (e.g., cysts, fibroadenomas)
Cancer
Diagnosis
History
Physical examination
Mammogram/ultrasound
Core biopsy
Treatment
Observation (for benign, stable masses)
Aspiration (for symptomatic or changing cysts)
Excisional biopsy (for symptomatic, changing masses, or core biopsy discordance)
Lumpectomy or mastectomy (for breast cancer)

CALCIFICATIONS

Calcifications of the breast are findings unique to the mammogram. Unless they are associated with other clinical findings, they are not detectable by the patient or the clinician. However, the finding of calcifications in the breast does warrant a clinical examination.

Like breast masses, calcifications have unique characteristics that can make them suspicious or benign.[8] They also have behaviors (stability or changes) that may raise or lower suspicions for breast cancer. As with masses, the preferred mode of biopsy for calcifications is core biopsy. Calcifications are biopsied using a special mammographic machine to obtain a stereotactic biopsy.[9] Excisional biopsy using wire localization is reserved for equivocal cores or calcifications not amenable to stereotactic core biopsy. In addition, calcifications may be followed without surgical intervention if they have benign features, show stability over time, or have benign histology on core biopsy.[10,11]

Table 7-6 summarizes the common causes, diagnosis, and treatment of calcifications.

SPECIAL SITUATIONS

THE PREGNANT FEMALE

The breast cancer survivor who is now a pregnant woman may present with all of the previously discussed problems. Unfortunately, breast cancer (primary or recurrence) can also present during pregnancy and lactation. It is said that breast cancer presenting during these periods is particularly virulent, most likely because it often presents at a later stage because of a delay in diagnosis. First, the breast during pregnancy and lactation can mask or confuse

TABLE 7-6 Calcifications: A Summary

Common Causes
Benign causes
Cancer
Diagnosis
History
Physical examination
Mammogram/ultrasound
Stereotactic core biopsy (for suspicious calcifications)
Excisional biopsy with wire localization (when stereotactic biopsy cannot be performed or for core biopsy discordance)
Treatment
Observation for benign calcifications
Lumpectomy or mastectomy for cancer

the clinical picture. Second, signs and symptoms of cancer are often erroneously attributed to these physiological states. Finally, fear of adversely affecting the pregnancy may cause a delay in performing an appropriate workup, including breast imaging and biopsy. Signs and symptoms in the breast of a pregnant or lactating woman should be as vigorously approached as when they are detected in her nonpregnant counterparts.

THE MALE BREAST

You may be providing survivorship care to men who have had breast cancer. Although such cases are rare—accounting for only 1% of all breast cancers—men do get breast cancer. It should not be considered normal for men to have any of the symptoms that have been described for women. Like women who present with complaints or abnormal clinical findings, men deserve and warrant a thorough breast workup, including breast imaging especially if he has had personal history of breast cancer. Genetics evaluation should also be considered for men with a history of breast cancer.[12,13]

Frequently Asked Questions

1. ***I just had a mammogram. Why do I need a new one now?***

   Mammograms that are obtained more than 3 months prior to a presenting problem should be considered old. In addition, a diagnostic mammogram complements the workup with additional views, ultrasounds, and other imaging modalities, as needed.

2. ***I have already had breast cancer, so why do I have to be concerned about benign breast disease?***

   It is appropriate to evaluate all breast abnormalities that are new to rule out the presence of local recurrence of the disease.

3. ***Should I see a breast surgeon before I get any workup or biopsy for benign breast disease?***

   Obtaining a diagnostic mammographic workup and even biopsy is appropriate and preferable, in that these measures facilitate the care of the patient should she need the services of a surgeon. They also may make the trip to the breast surgeon's office unnecessary.

4. ***Isn't it better and safer to have an excisional biopsy than a core biopsy?***

   Core biopsy is preferable to excisional biopsy because it is minimally invasive and maintains the integrity of the breast should further treatment be needed. Core biopsy is safe and does not cause the spread of cancer to other parts of the breast, lymph nodes, or other parts of the body.

5. ***My breast infection went away after I took antibiotics, so why do I need a mammogram now?***

   Infections in the breast are not normal; they should always be viewed with suspicion and their causes explained. Mammographic workups should always be standard after any infection.

REFERENCES

1. Breastcancer.org. Breast cancer symptoms and diagnosis [Web page]. Available at: http://www.breastcancer.org/symptoms. Accessed September 21, 2009.
2. Ibitoye BO, Adetiloye VA, Aremu AA. The appearance of benign breast diseases on ultrasound. *Niger J Med.* 2006;15(4):421–426.
3. Graf O, Helbich TH, Hopf G, et al. Probably benign breast masses at US: is follow-up an acceptable alternative to biopsy? *Radiology.* 2007;244(1):87–93.
4. Kollur SM, El Hag IA. FNA of breast fibroadenoma: observer variability and review of cytomorphology with cytohistological correlation. *Cyto-pathology.* 2006;17(5):239–244.
5. Breastcancer.org. Available at: http://www.breastcancer.org/symptoms/understand_bc/faq_symp/pain.jsp. Accessed September 22. 2009.
6. Rissanen T, Reinikainen H, Apaja-Sarkkinen M. Breast sonography in localizing the cause of nipple discharge: comparison with galactography in 52 patients. *J Ultrasound Med.* 2007;26(8):1031–1039.
7. Richards T, Hunt A, Courtney S, Umeh H. Nipple discharge: a sign of breast cancer? *Ann R Coll Surg Engl.* 2007;89(2):124–126.
8. Holcomb SS. Understanding mammogram microcalcifications. *Nurse Pract.* 2007;32(6):12–15.
9. Kikuchi M, Tsunoda-Shimizu H, Kawasaki T, et al. Indications for stereotactically guided vacuum-assisted breast biopsy for patients with category 3 microcalcifications. *Breast Cancer.* 2007;14(3):285–291.

10. Tse GM, Tan PH, Cheung HS, et al. Intermediate to highly suspicious calcifications in breast lesions: a radio-pathology correlation. *Breast Cancer Res Treat.* 2008;110(1):1–7.
11. Liu X, Inciardi M, Bradley JP, et al. Microcalcifications of the breast: size matters. A mammographic–histologic correlation study. *Pathologica.* 2007;99(1):5–10.
12. Narula HS, Carolson HE. Gynecomastia. *Endocrinology Metab Clinic North Am.* 2007:36(2):497–519.
13. Hines SL, Tan WW, Yasrebi M, et al. The role of mammography in male patients with breast symptoms. *Mayo Clinic Proc.* 2007;82(3):297–300.

CHAPTER 8

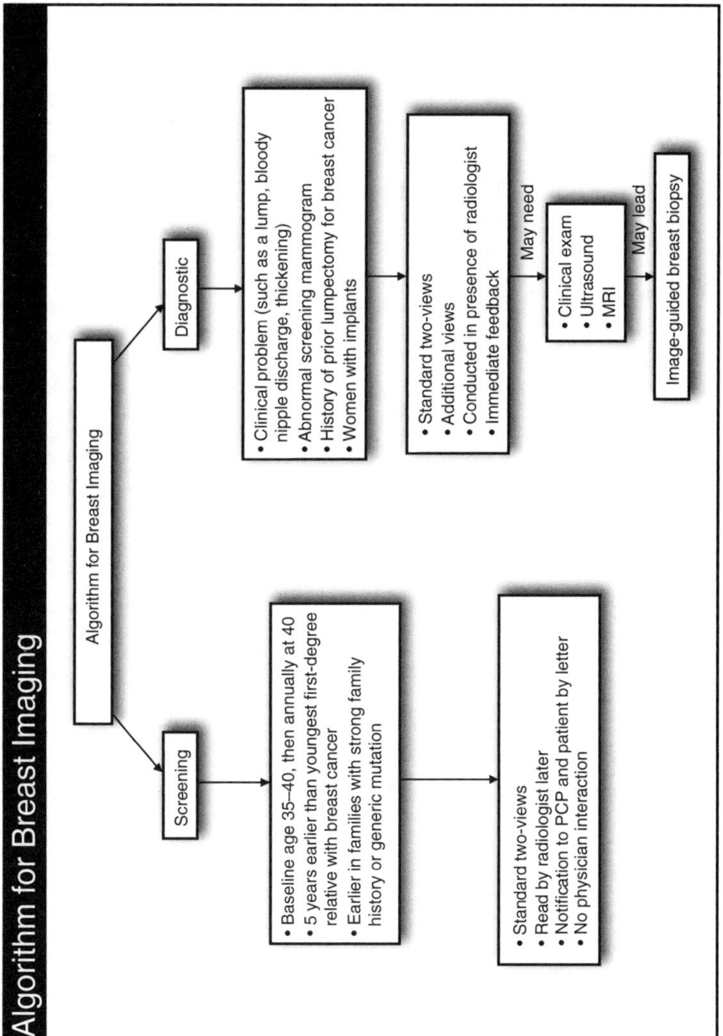
Algorithm for Breast Imaging
Algorithm for Breast Imaging
Screening
Diagnostic
• Baseline age 35–40, then annually at 40
• 5 years earlier than youngest first-degree relative with breast cancer
• Earlier in families with strong family history or generic mutation
• Standard two-views
• Read by radiologist later
• Notification to PCP and patient by letter
• No physician interaction
• Clinical problem (such as a lump, bloody nipple discharge, thickening)
• Abnormal screening mammogram
• History of prior lumpectomy for breast cancer
• Women with implants
• Standard two-views
• Additional views
• Conducted in presence of radiologist
• Immediate feedback
May need
• Clinical exam
• Ultrasound
• MRI
May lead
Image-guided breast biopsy

CHAPTER 8

Diagnostic Evaluation/Image-Guided Biopsies

Nagi F. Khouri, MD

What you need to know:

Screening mammography has reduced breast cancer mortality by 30% and in some studies by as much as 60% for women who have it performed annually.

Screening mammography criteria for you to follow with your patients are as follows:

- ▶ Women age 40 years and older should have it done annually; women age 80 years and older can have it done every other year.
- ▶ Women who have a first-degree relative diagnosed with breast cancer should begin mammography 5 years prior to the age their relative was at time of diagnosis.
- ▶ Women with several first-degree relatives diagnosed with breast cancer should begin mammography 10 years prior to the youngest age of their relative at time of diagnosis; they may also need genetic counseling. Mammographic screening is rarely used

for women younger than 30 years of age. Ultrasound is more commonly used for women in this age group for evaluation of a problem such as a lump.

Approximately 5% to 15% of women having a screening mammogram will be called back for additional imaging. Most of the time the findings of additional imaging will be benign.

Digital mammography is the newest form of breast-imaging technology for screening. If available, it would be the preferred modality. It is especially beneficial for your patients who have dense breasts and who are at high risk for developing breast cancer.

Be specific and accurate in describing breast symptoms or problems when referring a patient for diagnostic-imaging evaluation. Whenever possible, provide the patient with the necessary referrals so that all investigations can be carried out. This may require additional imaging studies and tests such as ultrasound, core biopsy, or both.

Breast ultrasound is beneficial as an adjunct imaging tool. It can define the extent of disease and differentiate solid masses (benign and malignant) from liquid-filled masses (cysts). Ultrasound is also useful in evaluating causes of nipple discharge.

Breast MRI is highly sensitive (90%) but not very specific (70%) and is less helpful in evaluating ductal carcinoma in situ (DCIS). It is useful for assessing multicentricity, multifocality, contralateral breast disease, axillary adenopathy, and tumor response to neoadjuvant chemotherapy. It is also used for adjunct screening for patients with BRCA1 and BRCA2 mutations and women with greater than a 20% lifetime risk for breast cancer.

A percutaneous image-guided biopsy is recommended whenever possible. More than 90% of breast biopsies can be obtained in a minimally invasive manner without an incision or general anesthesia and still provide an accurate histopathologic diagnosis. However, they should be performed by a trained healthcare provider who specializes in these procedures.

What your patient needs to know:

Mammography remains the best method for early detection of breast cancer. Mammograms do not prevent breast cancer. Their use is intended to detect breast cancer at its earliest possible stage when it is easiest to treat and survival can be at its highest.

Women who are compliant with their annual screening mammograms have a higher probability of early diagnosis and survival according to studies that confirm that the use of screening mammograms has reduced breast cancer mortality by 30% to 60%.

Women should not panic if they are called back for additional imaging following a screening mammogram. Most will learn that the final outcome is benign.

Other forms of breast imaging, such as ultrasound, are not to be used as a substitute for screening mammograms. They are designed as adjunct imaging when needed and recommended.

The quality of the mammogram and its accuracy in identifying breast cancer correlate to some degree with the thoroughness the mammography technologist uses in ensuring that the breast is adequately compressed and that the maximal amount of breast tissue is captured on the image.

The radiologist who specializes in breast imaging usually makes the decision when additional imaging is needed, such as ultrasound or breast MRI.

Women should not attempt to read their own mammograms or ultrasound images.

They should go to a facility that is reputable and has shown interest in specializing in breast imaging.

If your patient has not received a copy of her results, she should call the facility and request them. All women and their ordering physicians are to receive written copies of their results.

BENEFITS OF MAMMOGRAPHIC SCREENING

Randomized clinical trials performed over the last 40 years have shown a mortality reduction from breast cancer of approximately 30% in women offered screening mammography. It is very likely that the decrease in mortality attributable to screening mammography carried out in the community may be underestimated. There are estimates from Sweden that the mortality reduction from breast cancer is more on the order of 50% to 60%, attributed to early detection with mammography.[1,2] Why the difference? Many factors could account for this:

- Marked improvement in mammographic technique and interpretation since the controlled clinical trials were carried out

- Issues of compliance (in the U.S. studies, as many as 30% of patients invited to be in the study group did not show up for all their screening studies and have yet to be included in the final count)
- Number of screening rounds, length of follow-up, and length of screening intervals. All play a role in underestimating the benefits of mammography when compared to performance of annual mammography, every year, for a lifetime.

Although the benefits from screening mammography have repeatedly been contested since the early studies in the 1960s, the general consensus is that mammographic screening is beneficial in significantly reducing mortality related to breast cancer.

Since screening mammography was adopted on a widespread basis by physicians and women in the United States in the early 1990s, the mortality from breast cancer has dropped about 25% overall, mostly as a result of early detection with use of mammography.

WHO IS AT RISK FOR DEVELOPING BREAST CANCER?

More than 70% of breast cancers occur in women who have absolutely no identifiable risk factor other than being a woman and increasing in age. Breast cancer affects women predominantly after the age of 40. Less than 5% of breast cancers in developed countries occur in women younger than the age of 40. This may be different in other parts of the world where breast cancer incidence is not insignificant in younger women.

Family history of breast cancer in a first-degree relative or in multiple family members represents a significant added risk. In addition, 5% to 10% of breast cancers result from an inherited mutation, only few of which have been identified so far, such as the BRCA1 and BRCA2 genes. In such families the risk for developing breast cancer is high and may be on the order of 60% to 80%. Not infrequently in these families, the breast cancers develop at younger ages.

Hormonal factors such as early menarche and late menopause as well as late first pregnancy (after age 35) also affect breast cancer risk. Prolonged use of hormonal replacement therapy has been associated with an increased risk for breast cancer. The discontinuation of hormonal therapy in 2002 by many women following the discovery of this associated risk, for example, resulted in a lower incidence of breast cancer in 2003.

Women who have had prior breast biopsies that revealed proliferative changes are at higher risk for breast cancer; those with atypical cells found by pathology are at even higher risk.

Women who have developed cancer in one of their breasts are at higher risk for the development of another cancer in that same breast or in the contralateral breast.

RECOMMENDATIONS FOR MAMMOGRAPHIC SCREENING

It is recommended that all women older than age 40 have mammographic screening every year. For women older than 80, for whom the incidence of breast cancer starts to decrease, every other year may be adequate.

For women who have at least a first-degree relative with breast cancer, it is generally recommended that they start screening 5 years before the age at which the youngest family member was diagnosed with breast cancer. In families in which there are several members with breast cancer, including first-degree relatives, as well as in families with a genetic mutation, it is recommended that mammographic screening start 10 years before the age of diagnosis of the youngest family member with breast cancer.

It is clearly established that women whose cancer is localized to the breast have much better outcomes than those whose cancer has spread regionally to the lymph nodes or more distantly to metastatic sites. Even in patients with localized disease, the smaller the tumor, the better the outcome. A woman with a 1-cm breast malignancy has a much better prognosis than one with a 3-cm malignancy, with a 90% chance of being cured versus a 50% to 60% chance of being cured, respectively.

SCREENING MAMMOGRAPHY VERSUS DIAGNOSTIC MAMMOGRAPHY

When referring a patient for a mammogram, it is extremely important to decide whether the patient should be referred for a screening or diagnostic mammogram, as these are conducted differently.

A screening mammogram is an x-ray examination of the breasts of asymptomatic women in an attempt to detect abnormal lesions of the breasts when they are small and nonpalpable. Women complaining of vague bilateral breast pain qualify for a screening mammogram. Generally a screening mammogram is conducted without a physician on site. Rarely will the films be evaluated while the patient is at the facility, although the films are reviewed immediately for quality. The patients leave the facility and receive a letter in the mail a few days later informing them of the results of the examination. Five percent to 15% of patients may be called for additional imaging to evaluate an area of questionable or definite abnormality. Most of these patients will have a negative final outcome.

Conversely, a diagnostic mammogram is an examination used to evaluate a patient with a breast mass or breast masses as well as other breast signs or symptoms such as spontaneous nipple discharge, skin change, thickening, or nipple retraction. A diagnostic mammogram also includes women who are asked to return after the screening mammogram for further diagnostic imaging, women whose breast cancers were treated with breast conservation, and women with implants. The diagnostic examination is conducted in the presence of the radiologist who is monitoring the study, and the results are conveyed directly to the patient.

DIGITAL MAMMOGRAPHY VERSUS FILM SCREEN MAMMOGRAPHY

Digital mammography is the latest technology for x-ray imaging of the breasts. Results of the American College of Radiology (ACRIN) Digital Mammographic Imaging Screen Trial (DMIST) study published in 2005 comparing digital and film mammography have shown that digital mammography is more sensitive for the detection of breast cancer in women younger than 50 years, women with mammographically dense breasts, and premenopausal or perimenopausal women.[3] In addition, digital technology allows the use of new applications that are not available for analog mammography, which include digital subtraction angiography, tomosynthesis (cross-sectional imaging), computer-aided detection (the equivalent of double reading), and electronic storage and transmission. The greatest impediment to the wide use of digital mammography is its cost. In 2006, less than 10% of the mammographic units in the United States were digital units. It will be several years before digital mammographic units will outnumber analog mammographic units.

There is no doubt that although mammography has its own limitations, whether digital or analog, we all depend on the technical quality of the mammogram and the expertise of the physician who is interpreting the study. Proper positioning and compression of the breasts, and proper density of the films are the technical components that determine whether a cancer is detectable on the image. Since the introduction in 1992 of the Mammography Quality Standards Act (MQSA), there has been an improvement in the quality of mammograms. This is not, however, uniform in clinical practice. Similarly, the expertise of the interpreting physician is essential for the detection of the early and subtle cancers. Women are encouraged to get their mammograms at facilities that have demonstrated commitment to high-quality breast imaging and interpretation.

COMMUNICATIONS IN BREAST IMAGING

When referring a patient for a diagnostic evaluation, it is extremely important to be specific and accurate in describing the problem.

If the patient is referred for the evaluation of a focal abnormality in the breast such as a lump, one should describe the location of the abnormality by referring to the o'clock position on the breast and the number of centimeters from the nipple (actually measured with a ruler and not estimated).

If the patient is being referred for the evaluation of a discharge, one should note whether the discharge is spontaneous; unilateral or bilateral; from a single opening or multiple openings; and whether it is bloody, brownish, watery, mucoid, milky, or greenish.

BREAST ULTRASOUND

Breast ultrasound is an extremely important adjunct to mammographic imaging.[4] Indications for breast ultrasound include characterization of a palpable or mammographically detected mass—that is, whether it is a solid mass or a cyst. If the mass does not meet the criteria to be called a cyst, ultrasound aids in characterization by delineating the following: complex cyst; abscess; and benign-appearing, malignant-appearing, or indeterminate-appearing mass.

Ultrasound is a necessary test for the evaluation of a definite lump or a question of a lump, irrespective of the age of the patient.

In the event of a mass being suspected or diagnosed to be a cancer, ultrasound is very helpful in delineating the extent of the disease within the breast immediately around the malignancy as well as evaluating the breast for multicentricity that is the presence of foci of cancer in the other quadrants of the breast. Breast ultrasound is also used to screen the contralateral breast for unsuspected malignancy (2% to 3% incidence).

In the presence of cancer, ultrasound evaluation of the axilla is carried out. If abnormal lymph nodes are detected, they can be biopsied percutaneously, usually by fine-needle aspiration (FNA).

Breast ultrasound is also used for the evaluation of nipple discharge when arising from a single opening (watery, mucoid, or bloody). In many instances an intraductal lesion may be seen.

Breast ultrasound is the primary modality for evaluating patients younger than age 30 who are referred for the evaluation of a lump. Mammography is rarely performed in patients younger than age 30.

Breast ultrasound screening is currently being evaluated.[5] Preliminary studies have shown that ultrasound screening will yield three cancers per 1000 screenings in high-risk individuals, nonpalpable and nonmammographically visible. More than 75% of these cancers have been stage 1. The problem with breast ultrasound is that it is operator dependent, physician intensive, and not reimbursed by insurance.

Finally, ultrasound is used to help perform image-guided percutaneous biopsy procedures.

BREAST MRI

Breast magnetic resonance imaging (MRI) has evolved as an extremely helpful tool for the evaluation of breast diseases.[6] It is extremely sensitive for the detection of invasive carcinoma of the breast, with sensitivity exceeding 90% and specificity of approximately 70%. It is less sensitive for ductal carcinoma in situ (DCIS). Current cancer-related indications for breast MRI include the following:

- Lesion characterization of proven or suspected cancer and delineation of extent of disease, including multifocality (within the same quadrant), multicentricity (cancer in other quadrants), and evaluation of the contralateral breast. Breast MRI may be considered if breast conservation surgery is very likely and there are concerns regarding the extent of the cancer.
- Axillary adenopathy proven to be caused by epithelial malignancy with a negative mammogram. MRI is helpful to identify the specific location of the primary tumor inside the breast.
- Grossly positive margins following lumpectomy with no preoperative MRI
- Monitoring response to neoadjuvant chemotherapy for patients with locally advanced breast cancer
- Suspicion of recurrent disease versus scar

Although the sensitivity of MRI is high for invasive carcinoma, false negatives may be seen with DCIS and invasive lobular cancer, and, occasionally, with tubular carcinoma. In addition, there are a number of instances of false-positive MRI studies such as with fibrocystic change, proliferative changes, fibroadenoma, papilloma, and sclerosing adenosis.

Breast MRI screening is increasingly likely to be used for high-risk individuals, such as patients with a known mutation (i.e., BRCA1 and BRCA2) and for individuals having multiple family members with a history of breast cancer without a mutation demonstrated or with lifetime risk greater than 20%. Breast MRI screening is not recommended for the general population of asymptomatic women.

If a suspicious lesion is detected on MRI that is not recognizable on the standard studies and does not correspond to anything visible on the mammogram, then a second-look ultrasound is recommended, directed to the area of concern. If visible, the lesion may be biopsied under ultrasound guidance; if not, it may need to be biopsied under MRI guidance. In addition, breast MRI is used for the evaluation of the augmented breast for implant integrity.

IMAGE-GUIDED BREAST BIOPSY

Percutaneous image-guided breast biopsies (ultrasound-guided, stereotactically guided, or MRI-guided biopsies) have almost totally replaced surgical excision for biopsy of a lesion from the breast.[7] The advantages are that the percutaneous image-guided biopsies are as accurate as surgical biopsies (with few exceptions), they are quick to perform, and they do not result in any scarring of the breasts. These procedures are very well tolerated and less expensive than surgical biopsy. If a diagnosis of benign disease is determined, then the lesion can be left alone and just simply monitored by periodic imaging. If the lesion is found to be malignant, then the patient can be spared a surgical biopsy and can go to a single, definitive surgical procedure.

If the lesion is visible under ultrasound, then it is easiest to biopsy under ultrasound guidance. If the lesion is not visible on ultrasound, which is most frequently the case with microcalcifications, then it would be biopsied under stereotactic guidance. If the lesion is detected only on MRI, even after a second-look ultrasound, then it may need to be biopsied using MRI guidance.

Whenever an image-guided biopsy of the breast is performed, the radiologist must make a statement whether the lesion was adequately and accurately sampled and whether the pathology and the imaging findings are concordant. If these are not concordant, then a recommendation to repeat the biopsy or resect the lesion should be made.

There are a few pathological findings on needle biopsy that are considered insufficient in that they may underestimate the disease process. These are atypical ductal hyperplasia, atypical lobular hyperplasia, and lobular carcinoma in situ. In those instances, surgical excision of the biopsy site is necessary. In more than 25% of cases with atypical cells, a more serious problem is discovered such as carcinoma in situ or invasive carcinoma. Any atypia on core biopsy should be followed by surgical excision.

The management of a diagnosis of papilloma on needle biopsy is controversial. There are significant instances in which surgical biopsy followed a diagnosis of papilloma and yielded, in addition, a diagnosis of DCIS. Some doctors prefer to resect all papillomas diagnosed by core biopsy; others are selective.

Finally, a diagnosis of a radial scar on core biopsy is considered insufficient, and surgical excision is warranted.

Most of the time an accurate diagnosis is made by needle biopsy indicating the presence of specific or nonspecific benign disease or of malignancy.

Frequently Asked Questions

1. ***My patient prefers to have ultrasound rather than mammogram for screening. Is this appropriate and adequate for evaluating and identifying early-stage breast cancer?***

   Mammography remains the gold standard for screening for breast cancer. Ultrasound is to be used as an adjunct tool for a breast evaluation. It is more appropriate for identifying and differentiating solid masses from cysts. Therefore, encourage your patient to continue to have annual mammograms for screening.

2. ***My patient complains that mammograms hurt too much and therefore declines to get her screening annually. What does Johns Hopkins tell patients to promote compliance with screening?***

   We tell them that mammography is a screening test that takes only a few minutes. They are welcome to take over-the-counter analgesics prior to testing if their breasts are extremely sensitive. We reiterate the value of mammography in early detection of breast cancer. It is also helpful to explain why the compression is so tight—to be able to see through the breast tissue and provide an accurate reading of the images.

3. ***If my patient is in her 20s and has a lump, is mammography the test that should be ordered for evaluation?***

Breast tissue in young women is dense, and mammography may not be the ideal method of evaluation in these women. It is also more sensitive to radiation. It is more common to use ultrasound for evaluating women in this age group. To facilitate the diagnostic evaluation, be specific in your referral documentation as to the patient's symptoms/clinical findings and request that the radiologist in breast imaging determine the most appropriate method of diagnostic evaluation rather than specifying to the radiologist which tests you want done.

4. ***I have routinely sent patients to a breast surgeon when I palpate a lump. Is this an appropriate referral process?***

It is better to get a diagnosis before sending your patient to a surgeon. Sending your patient to a surgeon also increases her anxiety because she assumes she will need an operation. Direct her instead to a breast-imaging facility for diagnostic evaluation, keeping in mind that more than 90% of biopsies can be done in breast-imaging settings as core biopsies, without the need for an incision or general anesthesia. This technique is better for the patient and provides accurate information.

5. ***Is digital mammography really superior to traditional analog film mammography?***

   Yes, it is. When you look at the images side by side, you can really see the difference between them. The clarity of digital mammography is impressive, and it is especially helpful for women who are at high risk and for women with dense breasts. Although only a small percentage of breast-imaging facilities currently have digital mammography, in the coming years more will adopt it, making it more readily available for your patients.

REFERENCES

1. Feig SA. Effect of screening mammography on population mortality from breast carcinoma. *Cancer.* 2002;95: 451–457.
2. Duffy SW, Tabar L, Chen H-H, et al. The impact of organized mammography service screening on breast carcinoma mortality in seven Swedish counties: a collaborative evaluation. *Cancer.* 2002;95:458–469.

3. National Cancer Institute. Clinical trials (PDQ): randomized screening and diagnostic study of digital mammography versus screen-film mammography in the detection of breast cancer in women [Web page]. Available at: http://www.cancer.gov/clinicaltrials/ACRIN-6652. Accessed October 23, 2009.
4. Mendelson EB. Problem solving ultrasound. *Radiol Clin N Am.* 2004;42:909–918.
5. Berg WA. Supplemental screening sonography in dense breasts. *Radiol Clin N Am.* 2004;42:845–852.
6. Lee CH. Problem solving MR imaging of the breast. *Radiol Clin N Am.* 2004;425:919–934.
7. Fajardo LL, Pisano ED, Caudry DJ, et al. Stereotactic and sonographic large core biopsy of a lone palpable breast lesion: results of the Radiologic Diagnostic Oncology Group V study. *Acad Radiol.* 2004;11:293–308.

CHAPTER 9

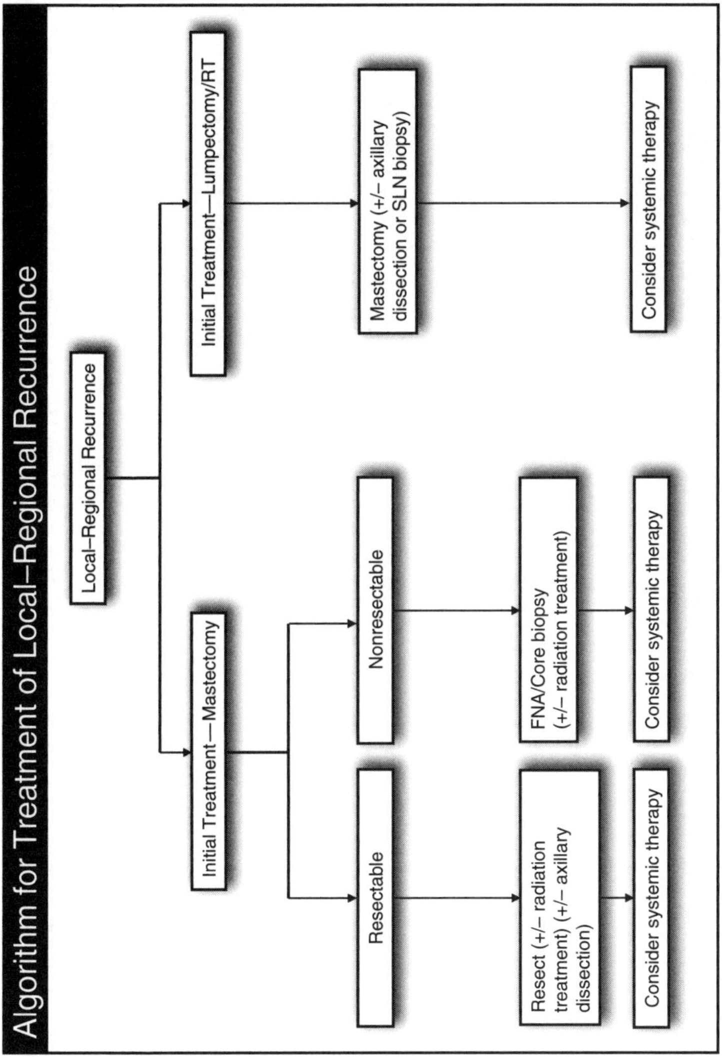
Algorithm for Treatment of Local–Regional Recurrence
Local–Regional Recurrence
Initial Treatment—Mastectomy
Initial Treatment—Lumpectomy/RT
Resectable
Nonresectable
Mastectomy (+/– axillary dissection or SLN biopsy)
Resect (+/– radiation treatment) (+/– axillary dissection)
FNA/Core biopsy (+/– radiation treatment)
Consider systemic therapy
Consider systemic therapy
Consider systemic therapy

CHAPTER 9

Algorithm for Treatment of Systemic Disease

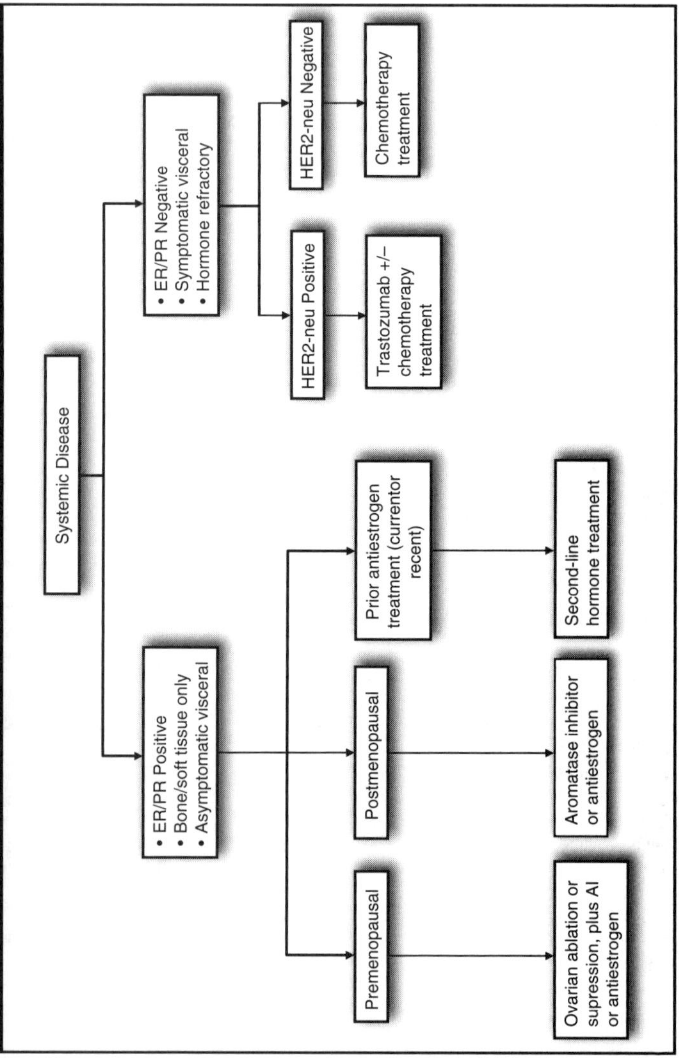

CHAPTER 9

The Diagnosis and Management of Recurrent and Metastatic Breast Cancer

Theodore N. Tsangaris, MD

What you need to know:

Local recurrence can be treated but should be considered a predictor of systemic disease and warrants consideration of systemic therapy.

The majority of time a local recurrence will declare itself during the time period that the patient is still being managed by her oncology specialists.

What your patient needs to know:

Having routine scans and tumor markers does not result in better clinical outcomes for a patient who has been diagnosed with metastatic breast cancer. The timing of identifying the disease does not have a direct bearing on her survival.

A diagnosis of metastatic breast cancer is devastating, but currently treatable, usually for multiple years.

The disease is treated like a chronic condition with the goal of keeping the disease stable and quality of life maintained for as long as possible.

Expensive screening tests and imaging are not appropriate for most women and do not improve survival from breast cancer.

Although a mammogram may have missed detecting the patient's breast cancer, mammograms are still the best screening tool for monitoring the breasts.

INTRODUCTION

Breast cancer is the most common malignancy in women. It is estimated that approximately 192,370 women will be newly diagnosed with invasive breast cancer in the United States in 2009. Additionally, 1,910 men will be diagnosed. Nearly 45,000 individuals will be diagnosed with ductal carcinoma in situ (DCIS), the most common type of noninvasive breast cancer, as well. Cancer of the breast is the second leading cause of cancer death in women after lung cancer. More than 40,000 women in the United States die each year of the disease.[1] Although the incidence of breast cancer continues to increase, mortality has been decreasing. In addition to the advances in screening and adjuvant therapy, this trend has been driven by a relatively recent (albeit modest) decrease in the rate of death from breast cancer. Nevertheless, however encouraging our treatment advances against the disease might be, women will still present with locally recurrent and metastatic disease.

Because of the greater use of breast-conserving surgery as the primary local therapy for breast cancer, clinicians can expect to see an increase in cases involving locally recurrent disease. Surgery offers an opportunity to decrease these ipsilateral breast tumor recurrences. However, systemic therapy in addition to local therapy is warranted for many of these individuals.

By contrast, metastatic disease is almost always not curable. The main goals of treatment of these patients are to control the disease, improve quality of life, and prolong life. Currently there are no absolute treatment approaches that work for all women. Generalized recommendations should be tailored to the patient and her individual circumstances. Clinical studies are defining the roles of endocrine therapy, chemotherapy, biologic therapy, and other novel approaches for treating metastatic disease.

SURVEILLANCE

In recent years, diagnostic testing for breast cancer patients has become more widely available. Traditionally, breast cancer follow-up has employed a conservative approach based on clinical examination and mammography. There is, however, marked variation in practice patterns, which can significantly affect the cost of delivering breast care. Equally important is the fact that excess or abuse of available diagnostic tools has never been shown to improve disease-free or overall survival rates.

Table 9-1 summarizes the current screening recommendations for breast cancer surveillance.

TABLE 9-1 Recommendations for Breast Cancer Surveillance

History and Physical Examination
By specialist or shared with PCP
Every 3 to 4 months for 3 years
Every 6 to 12 months for 2 years
Annually after 5 years
Mammography
New baseline: 6 to 12 months after definitive radiation therapy
Ipsilateral breast: every 6 months until stability is established, then annually
Contralateral breast: annually
Breast Self-Examination
Every month
Pelvic Examination
Routine yearly examination
Routine Blood Tests
No
Routine Imaging
No (includes computed tomography, positron-emission tomography, and magnetic resonance imaging)
Routine Tumor Markers
No

HISTORY AND PHYSICAL EXAMINATION

All women should have a careful history and physical examination every 3 to 4 months for the first 3 years after primary therapy, then every 6 to 12 months for the next 2 years, and then annually thereafter.

A word about examining the postlumpectomy and radiated breast is warranted here. In general, the same principles of technique apply as when examining a breast that has not been treated for cancer. Examining the treated breast in the same systematic way the clinician has developed in his or her practice for examining the normal breast is very important. However, the radiated breast will feel different than the non-irradiated breast. Initially after treatment, the skin will feel thicker and the breast parenchyma will be firmer. A residual mass or local distortion of the breast might be noted at the lumpectomy site. Over time, the breast will attempt to return to its prelumpectomy and radiation state. Although they may never be completely normal, after treatment most breasts will look and feel very similar to the nontreated breast.

It is important to acknowledge the patient's concern that the treated breast might be difficult to monitor during the immediate posttreatment period. Reassurance, patience, and encouragement will be very important to the patient's acceptance of and comfort level with the posttreatment breast. Relatively frequent examinations provide both the patient and the clinician the opportunity to compare notes and impressions on the progress of the treated breast. These visits are beneficial to the clinician and patient in accepting and surveying the breast. In rare cases, the irradiated breast never progresses favorably cosmetically. These patients will be more challenging to monitor and will need special understanding.

Finally, although subtle changes in the treated breast are appropriate, discrete abnormalities that progress are never normal and always warrant further investigation.

BREAST SELF-EXAMINATION

All women should be instructed on how to perform monthly breast self-examination (BSE).

MAMMOGRAPHY

Mammography should be initiated approximately 6 months after definitive radiation therapy for women treated with breast-conserving therapy. Subsequent mammograms should be obtained every 6 to 12 months while establishing stability. Annual mammograms should follow when stability is achieved.

COORDINATION OF CARE

Continuity of care for the patient with breast cancer is recommended and should be undertaken by a healthcare provider experienced in the surveillance of cancer patients and breast examination. Familiarity with and a level of comfort in the examination of the irradiated breast are very important. You may be the professional assuming follow-up care, provided you meet the aforementioned requirements. The nurse practitioner should be expected to achieve results similar to those delivered by a breast oncology specialist (surgeon or medical oncologist). A "shared-care" model of patient follow-up has been suggested and may be more appropriate, depending on the stage of disease and the requirements of long-term treatment such as adjuvant endocrine therapy. For patients still receiving hormonal therapy treatment, she may be seeing her medical oncologist annually and you also annually, so that every 6 months someone is evaluating her and monitoring her care.

PELVIC EXAMINATION

A regular annual gynecologic follow-up is recommended for all women. Patients on tamoxifen therapy should report any vaginal bleeding promptly given that they are at increased risk for developing endometrial cancer. Communication and coordination of care with her gynecologist is also helpful in that this healthcare provider is also assessing her for local recurrence of disease when performing a CBE. This doctor also has a role in assessing her endometrial health, with a special focus on patients who are receiving tamoxifen.

BREAST CANCER SURVEILLANCE TESTING: NOT RECOMMENDED

The following tests are not recommended for routine breast cancer surveillance: complete blood count (CBC), blood chemistries, chest x-rays, bone scans, ultrasounds of the liver, computed tomography (CT) scans, positron-emission tomography (PET) scans, breast magnetic resonance imaging (MRI), and breast cancer blood tumor markers (CA 15-3, CA 27.29, and carcinoembryonic antigen [CEA]).

LOCAL–REGIONAL RECURRENCE

IPSILATERAL BREAST TUMOR RECURRENCE

The use of breast-conserving therapy as the local treatment of choice for most early-stage breast cancers continues to increase. Studies suggest that patients who undergo such treatment have a 5% to 15% risk for ipsilateral breast tumor recurrence (IBTR). These recurrences are emotionally taxing to the patient and her healthcare providers but definitely treatable. Most women who have had lumpectomy and radiation are best treated with completion mastectomy. Simple reexcision of the recurrence may be appropriate in selected patients and under special circumstances.

The significance of an IBTR appears to go beyond the immediate problem and anxiety of treating the local recurrence. Meta-analysis suggests that an IBTR is not the instigator of a patient's demise but rather a prognosticator of future systemic disease. For this reason, strong consideration should be given to providing any patient who experiences an IBTR with systemic therapy in addition to treating the visible local disease.

CHEST WALL RECURRENCE

There is no question that local recurrence of cancer in the chest wall, after initial mastectomy, carries a far more ominous significance than an in-breast tumor recurrence after breast-conserving therapy. The active search for metastatic disease is appropriate and unfortunately often fruitful. Systemic therapy is often used in this scenario. The presence of other metastatic sites, disease-free interval, prior treatment history, and performance score are all important factors when considering the multidisciplinary approach to these patients.

Nothing is more devastating to a patient than uncontrolled local chest wall disease. Referral back to her breast surgeon and medical oncologist should be expedited. When possible, a breast surgeon will perform a local resection with clear margins and radiation therapy should be utilized. If complete resection with clear margins is not possible, then obtaining tissue through fine-needle aspiration (FNA) or core biopsy is important in facilitating systemic therapy. Incisional or partial resections should be avoided, as retained tumor at the surgical site can make healing difficult, if not impossible.

REGIONAL NODAL RECURRENCE

In the past, level I and II axillary dissection was performed with a lumpectomy, making resampling of the axilla for IBTR unnecessary and futile. However, the advent of the sentinel lymph node (SLN) biopsy as the standard of care has challenged this dogma. It may be appropriate to perform axillary dissection in IBTR for patients with a prior SLN biopsy. The more intriguing question may be whether it is appropriate to repeat SLN biopsy as a substitute for formal level I and II axillary dissection in these patients.

An increasing volume of experience reported in the literature has shown the success and accuracy of SLN biopsy for local recurrence of breast cancer after breast-conserving therapy. The absolute number of lymph nodes removed during the initial axillary sampling (which represents a surrogate marker for the extent of surgical manipulation and alteration of the lymph node basin) seems to be important when considering a repeat SLN biopsy. Studies suggest that reoperative SLN biopsy is more successful when fewer than 10 lymph nodes were removed in previous surgeries. Variation in the dye migration times and drainage pathways was also seen with increasing lymph node numbers. In addition to drainage to the ipsilateral axilla, lymphoscintigraphy revealed drainage to the internal mammary chain, interpectoral nodes, supraclavicular nodes, and contralateral axillary basin. For this reason, preoperative lymphoscintigraphy should be used before any approach to the axilla. However, as in cases of primary breast cancer, restraint should be implemented when sampling of the axilla will not influence subsequent systemic treatment or radiation therapy.

Internal mammary and supraclavicular lymph nodes are usually not addressed surgically. However, knowledge of their involvement could be important in determining the patient's prognosis and planning for systemic therapy and radiotherapy.

TREATMENT OF DISTANT METASTASES

The appearance of metastatic breast cancer is always devastating and almost never curable. You will be referring the patient back to her medical oncologist for management. Due to your relationship with the patient, you may choose to continue to see her at periodic intervals. Her treatment plan, however, will be established and should be shared with you. She may wish to rely on you for additional support. Yet even in light of that disease dynamic, clear goals exist for managing patients with metastatic breast cancer:

- Cure the disease (though rare).
- Improve overall survival.
- Improve time to progression.
- Improve symptoms related to the disease.
- Improve quality of life.

In reality, the main goals in the treatment of metastatic disease are to control the disease, improve the quality of life, and prolong life.

As with adjuvant treatment, the clinician dealing with recurrent and metastatic disease must assess the patient for prognostic and predictive factors. Prognostic factors include an estimation of outcome independent of systemic treatment. This would be reflected in factors such as (1) tumor biology, (2) site of disease, (3) extent of disease, (4) time to recurrence, and (5) prior therapy. Predictive factors would reflect a relative resistance or sensitivity to a specific therapy such as estrogen receptor (ER) status or HER2/neu status. In addition, patient characteristics should be considered, including age, menopausal status, and performance status (i.e., ability to perform daily activities of living). Finally, balancing toxicity and efficacy is always a concern for the patient and her healthcare team.

Clinical studies are constantly looking at the roles of endocrine therapy, chemotherapy, and biologic therapy in patients with metastatic breast cancer. Therapy options include the following:

- Endocrine therapies
- Chemotherapy
- Novel therapies
- Supportive therapy

These modalities will be discussed separately in further detail.

ENDOCRINE THERAPY

Approximately one third (67%) of patients with recurrent breast cancers will express estrogen receptors (ER) or progesterone receptors (PR). More than half of these women will benefit from interventions that modulate ER or reduce estrogen content. Therefore, endocrine intervention should be considered as first-line therapy in women with newly diagnosed hormone receptor-positive breast cancer.

A number of endocrine agents are currently available for use against metastatic breast cancer. They include the following classes of hormonal agents and other endocrine-based treatments:

- Selective estrogen receptor modulators (SERMS)
- Aromatase inhibitors (AIs)
- Estrogen receptor inhibitors
- Progesterone
- Ovarian ablation

Tamoxifen (a SERM) is effective in both premenopausal and postmenopausal women. Although tamoxifen has traditionally been the first-line treatment of choice for metastatic breast cancer, AIs' arrival on the scene has led them to challenge tamoxifen as the drug of choice in many situations. Several AIs have compared favorably with tamoxifen, even demonstrating some advantage compared with the latter drug. For instance, anastrozole, exemestane, and letrozole have all shown equivalence or superiority to tamoxifen in several studies in terms of both clinical response and time to progression. Of course, AIs are effective only in the absence of ovarian function. Therefore, in premenopausal women for whom tamoxifen is not appropriate, to reduce circulating estrogen the physician should prescribe ovarian suppression with or without an AI. Postmenopausal women should be placed on an AI.

Fulvestrant is a selective ER downregulator that acts as a pure antiestrogen. When administered intramuscularly on a monthly basis, it has been found to compare favorably to anastrozole in clinical trials; there are no significant differences in clinical response or time to progression for these two drugs. Fulvestrant has also been compared with tamoxifen as first-line therapy for metastatic breast cancer. Although the two drugs compared favorably with respect to time to progression and objective response, the clinical benefit was greater for tamoxifen.

The variations in the effectiveness of SERMs, AIs, and ER downregulators for particular patient groups merely emphasize the complexity of hormone therapy and the fact that there are several valid choices for therapy. In principle, the sequential use of hormone therapy is warranted. Studies are under way to examine the efficacy of combinations of agents such as anastrozol and fulvestrant relative to their efficacy as single-agent therapies.

CHEMOTHERAPY (NONENDOCRINE THERAPY)

Nonhormonal therapy may be considered for the following indications:

- Hormone-negative breast cancer
- Rapidly progressing visceral metastasis regardless of hormonal status
- Hormone-positive disease that is refractory to sequential endocrine therapy
- Short disease-free interval following adjuvant treatment

Several factors need to be considered when choosing chemotherapy for patients with metastatic breast cancer. First, the relative benefits and toxicities of the various options for the individual patient must be considered. There are multiple options of treatment to consider, including combination versus single-agent chemotherapy, the role of dose-intense or dose-dense therapy, and biologically targeted therapy. Of course, while choosing an appropriate therapy, quality of life issues must be kept in perspective.

Several single-agent chemotherapy options have been effective as first- or second-line therapy. Of the popular classes of agents, taxanes and anthracyclines have been the most effective. With the increased use of these drugs in the adjuvant setting, the patient with newly diagnosed metastatic disease presents the clinician with a therapeutic dilemma. If the patient has been treated with an anthracycline or taxane in the previous 6 to 12 months, it might be preferable to start treatment with a different class of drugs. However, if a longer time has passed since use of these agents, then retreatment with an anthracycline or taxane might be considered. The availability of new forms of anthracyclines, such as epirubicin and the liposomal anthracyclines, has decreased concerns about cardiotoxicity and made retreatment with this class of drug for metastatic disease more feasible.

The question of sequential, single-agent therapy versus combination chemotherapy for the treatment of metastatic breast cancer remains an important issue. Combination therapy seems to improve response rates and time to progression. However, these benefits must be weighed against the greater toxicity associated with the combination therapy. It has also been difficult to prove improved overall survival rates for particular combinations. The following classes of drugs are used as both single and combination therapies:

- Alkylating agents
- Antimetabolites
- Vinca alkaloids
- Anthracyclines
- Taxanes
- Nucleoside analogs

Part of the difficulty in determining the benefits of single-agent versus combination therapy is the comparison of "apples to oranges." Many studies have compared one agent with a combination of different agents rather than comparing the same agents either in sequence or in combination. A recent Eastern Cooperative Oncology Group study (ECOG 1193) did use a crossover design, which allowed for the direct comparison of sequential, single-agent treatment and combination therapy. The objective response and time to progression were better with the combination therapy, but no statistically significant difference in overall survival was noted for single-agent versus combination therapy. Also encountered, however, were increases in grade 3 and 4 toxicities.

The correct choice of single-agent versus combination therapy might ultimately rest with the clinical needs of the specific patient. If a significant response is needed clinically, then combination therapy would be warranted. If the concern is minimizing toxicity without compromising survival or quality of life, then sequential therapy could be more appropriate.

NOVEL THERAPIES

Novel therapies for metastatic disease include trastuzumab (Herceptin), lapatinib (Tykerb), and bevacizumab.

Trastuzumab, a humanized antibody, targets and binds to the human epidermal growth factor receptor 2 (EGFR-2; also known as HER2/neu) in tumor cells. HER2/neu is a tyrosine kinase transmembrane growth factor receptor that is localized to chromosome 17q. Amplification or overexpression of this receptor is seen in as many as 30% of patients with breast cancer; it is correlated with a worse survival as compared with HER2/neu-negative tumors. HER2/neu-positive tumors have increased cell proliferation, demonstrate increased cell migration, and are resistant to apoptosis. By downregulating the HER2/neu receptor and reducing tumor cell proliferation, trastuzumab is effective as a single agent when used as first-line therapy against HER2/neu-positive cancers.

Data also suggest that there are synergies between trastuzamab and certain chemotherapeutic agents such as cisplatin, docetaxel, thiotepa, and etoposide. Cardiotoxicity again is a concern with combination therapy consisting of trastuzumab and anthracyclines, but less so with the trastuzumab–paclitaxel combination. Ongoing trials investigating the combination of trastuzumab and liposomal anthracyclines have shown encouraging reductions in toxicity while maintaining promising response rates. In addition, trials exploring the flexibility of dosing trastuzamab and the continuation of trastuzamab after first-line therapy are also under way.

Lapatinib binds to intracellular ATP-binding sites of HER2/neu and EGFR (ErbB-1), blocking downstream signaling. This dual blockade may be more effective than the single-target inhibition provided by agents such as trastuzumab.

In a phase I trial of lapatinib and capecitabine, lapatinib was well tolerated and showed clinical activity. This drug has shown activity in trastuzumab-resistant breast cancer both in cell lines and in clinical trials.

Tumor growth is dependent on angiogenesis. Bevacizumab is a humanized monoclonal antibody directed against vascular endothelial growth factor (VEGF). It appears to have activity in patients with refractory metastatic breast cancer.

The emergence of new and novel treatments is an exciting and encouraging development for both patients and clinicians. Patients who would benefit from systemic therapy for metastatic breast cancer should be encouraged to participate in clinical trials when appropriate.

BISPHOSPHONATES

Pamidronate and zoledronic acid are drugs that bind to the bone matrix and reduce the number of adverse events associated with bone metastasis. They also prolong the time to the first event. Patients with bone disease and pain experience a clinically relevant analgesic effect when they take these drugs. Given this fact, bisphosphonates should be given in addition to hormone therapy or chemotherapy for patients with bone metastasis, or to patients with a reasonable expected survival. These drugs should be administered in conjunction with calcium and vitamin D.

Bisphosphonates are associated with a range of toxicities. Renal toxicities have been observed, for example, so good renal function with close monitoring of creatinine clearance is important in patients who take these drugs. Osteonecrosis of the jaw has also been reported during long-term use of bisphosphonates.

SURGERY

The role of the breast surgical oncologist or other surgical specialist in cases of distant metastatic disease is generally one of palliation. Although the decision to surgically intervene for palliation often has merit, the patient needs to understand that cure is rarely possible. The risks and benefits of any surgical intervention should be thoroughly explored by the patient and her healthcare team. Patients with isolated liver metastasis have traditionally been considered to have a poor prognosis, with median survival rates of less than 6 months. Several institutions have reported on the use of the surgical approach in these situations. In studies with limited numbers of patients, morbidity and mortality are relatively low with modest gains in survival. Factors that favor a better outcome for these patients are hormone status of tumor, histologic grade, number of other metastatic organ sites, performance scores, and time to developing initial liver metastasis. Again, although some have advocated metastasectomy in selected cases of isolated lesions with reported improved survival rates, these scenarios are the exception and should be rigorously scrutinized on a case-by-case basis. Newer studies are also raising the controversial question as to whether there is any benefit to performing a mastectomy to remove the primary source of the disease in situations in which the patient is diagnosed from the onset with stage IV breast cancer. However, more data are needed to determine whether this is of benefit from a survival perspective. For women with locally advanced disease that is causing pain, mastectomy is sometimes performed for local control.

RADIATION THERAPY

As for surgery, the role of radiation therapy (RT) for metastatic disease is largely one of palliation. Radiation therapy may be preferable to surgery in such cases, however, because of its ability to quickly achieve the desired effect on the disease and its avoidance of the morbidity associated with surgery. Brain metastases have increased in frequency, probably as a result of advances in palliative care. In patients with good performance scores and in the absence of multiple metastatic sites, intensified local treatment with systemic therapy appears to influence time to progression and overall survival.

The following are clinical situations for which surgery and/or radiation may provide significant palliation:

- Brain metastases
- Leptomeningeal disease
- Choroid metastases
- Pleural effusion
- Pericardial effusion
- Biliary obstruction

- Ureteral obstruction
- Impending pathologic fracture
- Pathologic fracture
- Cord compression
- Localized painful bone or soft-tissue disease
- Chest wall disease

In any case, the decision to perform surgery or administer radiation therapy for palliation should be undertaken only after careful consideration of the risks and benefits to the patient.

PALLIATIVE CARE

Statistics suggest that more than 85% of patients with advanced cancer will ultimately die of their disease. Although palliative care is now considered integral to the care of these patients, most patients are referred too late to get the full benefit of what is available. Unfortunately, many patients are never referred to palliative care at all. The World Health Organization (WHO) recommends that palliative care be initiated at the same time that therapy for disease is implemented.

The National Comprehensive Cancer Network (NCCN) Palliative Care Guidelines were developed to facilitate the integration of palliative care into oncology practice. Included in the guidelines are procedures for screening, assessment, intervention, reassessment, and after-death care. The needs of the family during this time and after death should also be addressed using these guidelines.

Frequently Asked Questions

1. ***I feel discomfort in my treated breast. Is this normal?***

   Discomfort after lumpectomy and radiation is normal. The frequency and intensity of the discomfort should diminish significantly with time but may last a lifetime.

2. ***Should I be getting a bone scan, CT scan, and blood test to see if my cancer is coming back?***

   Current recommendations are not to get expensive imaging and blood tests for routine screening. They have never been shown to improve survival.

3. ***Do I have to undergo a mastectomy after a local (in-breast) recurrence of my breast cancer?***

   Most women with in-breast recurrences will require mastectomy. Special exceptions may be made for women with small recurrences, long disease-free intervals, and the presence or absence of comorbidities.

4. ***Why do I need systemic therapy after mastectomy for a local recurrence?***

   A local recurrence is considered a predictor of systemic disease and warrants consideration of adjuvant therapy.

REFERENCE

1. National Cancer Institute. Breast cancer home page [Web page]. Available at: http://www.cancer.gov/cancertopics/types/breast. Accessed October 23, 2009.

FURTHER READING

Carlson RW, Allred DC, Anderson BO, et al. *NCCN clinical practice guidelines for breast cancer,* v.1.2007. Available at: http://www.nccn.org/professionals/physician_gls/f_guidelines.asp. Accessed October 23, 2009.

Fisher B, Anderson S, Fisher ER, et al. Significance of ipsilateral breast tumor recurrence after lumpectomy. *Lancet.* 1991;338(8763):327–331.

Gralow JR. Optimizing the treatment of metastatic breast cancer. *Breast Cancer Res Treat.* 2005;89:s9–s15.

Khatcheressian JL, Wolff AC, Smith TJ, et al. American Society of Clinical Oncology 2006 update of the breast cancer follow-up and management guidelines in the adjuvant setting. *J Clin Oncol.* 2006;24(31):5091–5097.

Levy MH, Back A, Benedetti C, et al. *NCCN clinical practice guidelines for palliative care,* v.1. 2006. Available at: http://www.nccn.org/professionals/physician_gls/f_guidelines.asp. Accessed October 23, 2009.

Luini A, Galimberti V, Gatti G, et al. The sentinel node biopsy after previous breast surgery: preliminary results on 543 patients treated at the European Institute of Oncology. *Breast Cancer Res Treat* 2005;89(2):159–163.

Taback B, Nguyen P, Hansen N, et al. Sentinel lymph node biopsy for local recurrence of breast cancer after breast-conserving therapy. *Ann Surg Oncol.* 2006;13(8):1099–1104.

Resources of Benefit—The American Cancer Society's Breast Cancer Network

American Cancer Society (ACS), National

800-ACS-2345
http://www.cancer.org/index.html

The American Cancer Society (ACS) is a nationwide, community-based organization with chartered divisions across the country. This Web site is the home page for information about clinical research trials funded by the ACS, including the Reach to Recovery program, which provides one-on-one support to newly diagnosed patients about the ACS's free programs such as Road to Recovery, I Can Cope, and Look Good, Feel Better. Also consider contacting your local ACS office for information and support.

American Society of Breast Surgeons

5950 Symphony Woods Road, Suite 212
Columbia, MD 21044
410-992-5470 or (toll free) 877-992-5470
Fax: 410-992-5472
contact@breastsurgeons.org
http://www.breastsurgeons.org

The American Society of Breast Surgeons was formed to encourage the study of breast surgery, to promote research and development of advanced surgical techniques, to improve standards of practice for breast surgery in the United States, and to serve as a forum for the exchange of ideas.

American Society of Clinical Oncology (ASCO)

http://www.asco.org

The American Society of Clinical Oncology (ASCO) is a nonprofit organization, founded in 1964, with overarching goals of improving cancer care and prevention and ensuring that all patients with cancer receive care of the highest quality. More than 23,000 oncology healthcare practitioners belong to ASCO, representing all oncology disciplines (medical, radiologic, and surgical oncology) and subspecialties.

As the world's leading professional organization representing physicians who treat people with cancer, ASCO is committed to advancing the education of oncologists and other oncology professionals, advocating for policies that provide access to high-quality cancer care, and supporting the clinical trials system and the need for increased clinical and translational research.

Amoena/Coloplast

http://www.thebreastcaresite.com

This is a Web site sponsored by Amoena/Coloplast. It provides educational information about breast health and breast cancer, including monthly articles and an Ask the Expert section.

Breastcancer.org

http://www.breastcancer.org

Breastcancer.org is a nonprofit organization dedicated to providing the most reliable, complete, and up-to-date information about breast cancer. Their mission is to help women and their loved ones make sense of the complex medical and personal information about breast cancer so they can make the best decisions for their lives.

Cancer Information Service of the National Cancer Institute

800-4-CANCER
http://www.cancer.gov

This organization provides information about all types of cancer including excellent information about breast cancer, what it is, how it is treated, and where various treatment options are provided. You can request free information by calling the toll-free number.

CancerNet—National Cancer Institute

900 Rockville Pike
Building #31, HSV2580, Room 10A046
Bethesda, MD 20892
800-422-6237
http://www.cancernet.nci.nih.gov

Provides patients with information about clinical trials that may be of benefit to them.

CenterWatch Clinical Trials Listing Service

581 Boylston Street, Suite 200
Boston, MA 02116
627-247-02116
http://www.centerwatch.com

Provides clinicians and patients with information about clinical trials available in their region.

The Johns Hopkins Avon Foundation Breast Center

443-287-2778 (BRST)
410-614-2853, Lillie D. Shockney's direct line
shockli@jhmi.edu
http://www.hopskinsbreastcenter.org

This breast center is one of the few comprehensive cancer centers in the country that offers state-of-the-art breast cancer diagnosis and treatment. A special feature online is *Artemis*, Hopkins' electronic breast cancer medical journal that you can subscribe to online for free. It is published online monthly and provides the most up-to-date information about the latest available research results and information related to the diagnosis and treatment of this disease. The Web site also has sections about diagnosis and treatment information, breast imaging, pathology and breast reconstruction, breast cancer patient bill of rights, and other valuable resource information. A new section recently added is dedicated to survivorship care.

Susan G. Komen for the Cure

National Helpline 800-IM-AWARE
http://www.komen.org

This is a national volunteer organization seeking to eradicate breast cancer as a life-threatening disease, working through local chapters and the Race for the Cure, it sponsors events in more than 110 cities. The foundation is the largest private funder of breast cancer research in the United States. The Komen Alliance is a comprehensive program for the research, education, diagnosis, and treatment of breast disease. You will find information on their Web site about their mission, the accomplishments they have achieved to date, how you can participate, grants they have funded, and calendar of national events, as well as other information. Komen is very big on education about the disease and on ensuring treatment for the underserved.

Mothers Supporting Daughters with Breast Cancer (MSDBC)

25235 Fox Chase Drive
Chestertown, MD 21620
410-778-1982
msdbc@verizon.net
http://www.mothersdaughters.org

This is a national, nonprofit organization dedicated to providing support to mothers who have daughters diagnosed with breast cancer. This organization offers a free "mother's handbook" and "daughter's companion booklet" that provides basic information about breast cancer and its treatment as well as some recommended constructive ways for mothers to provide support physically, emotionally, financially, and spiritually. The organization also "matches" mothers with mother volunteers across the country based on the daughter's (patient's) clinical picture, age at the time of diagnosis, and anticipated treatment plan.

National Comprehensive Cancer Network (NCCN)

http://www.nccn.org

The National Comprehensive Cancer Network (NCCN), a nonprofit alliance of 20 of the world's leading cancer centers, is dedicated to improving the quality and effectiveness of care provided to patients with cancer. Through the leadership and expertise of clinical professionals at NCCN member institutions, NCCN develops resources that present valuable information to the numerous stakeholders in the healthcare delivery system. As the arbiter of high-quality cancer care, NCCN promotes the importance of continuous quality improvement and recognizes the significance of creating clinical practice guidelines appropriate for use by patients, clinicians, and other healthcare decision makers. The primary goal of all NCCN initiatives is to improve the quality, effectiveness, and efficiency of oncology practice so patients can live better lives. NCCN offers a number of programs to give clinicians access to tools and knowledge that can help guide decision making in the management of cancer. Johns Hopkins is a member of this alliance. At the NCCN Web site you will find the Breast Cancer Treatment guidelines written out for clinicians as well as a patient-friendly set to give your patients. You can also obtain hard copies of these documents from your local ACS.

National Consortium of Breast Centers (NCBC)

P.O. Box 1334
Warsaw, IN 46581-1334

574-267-8058
Fax: 574-267-8268
wiggins@breastcare.org
http://www.breastcare.org or http://www.ncbcinc.org

The National Consortium of Breast Centers' (NCBC) mission and purpose, according to its bylaws and articles of incorporation, is "to promote excellence in breast health care for the general public through a network of diverse professionals dedicated to the active exchange of ideas and resources, including: (1) to serve as an informational resource and to provide support services to those rendering care to people with breast diseases through educational programs, newsletters, a national directory, and patient forums; (2) to encourage professionals to concentrate and specialize in activities related to breast disease; (3) to encourage the development of programs and centers that address breast disease and promote breast health; (4) to facilitate collaborative research opportunities on issues of breast health, and; (5) to develop a set of core measures to define, improve, and sustain quality standards in comprehensive breast programs and centers."

Johns Hopkins Breast Center faculty have been directly involved in chairing the National Consortium of Breast Centers Quality Initiative, designed to facilitate the development of national quality standards for the diagnosis and treatment of breast cancer. The NCBC provides through this initiative an opportunity to measure and assess quality of care. They also work to improve efficiency, effectiveness, and quality outcomes. Nurse practitioners, PCPs, and gynecologists are encouraged and welcome to attend the conferences. NCBC also offers a certification exam for nurses working in the field of breast care and breast cancer.

National Institutes of Health

http://www.clinicaltrials.gov

Provides clinicians and patients with information pertaining to clinical trials for each type of cancer.

Network of Strength (formerly known as the Y-Me National Breast Cancer Organization)

800-221-2141 (24-hour national hotline)
800-986-9505 (24-hour hotline in Spanish)
info@y-me.org
http://www.y-me.org or
http://www.networkofstrength.org

Network of Strength is committed to providing information and support to anyone who has been touched by breast cancer. The services listed on their Web site include a national hotline for women needing emotional support, a kid's corner, referral information for approved mammography facilities near you, public education workshops where you will find a listing of upcoming events, teen programs where you can order a video specifically for teenage girls to learn about breast cancer awareness, and a resource library that provides information about treatment modalities.

People Living with Cancer

http://www.plwc.org

People Living with Cancer, the patient information Web site of the American Society of Clinical Oncology (ASCO), is designed to help patients and families make informed healthcare decisions. The Web site provides information on more than 85 types of cancer, clinical trials, coping, side effects, a database to help you find an oncologist, patient support organizations, and more.

Society of Surgical Oncology (SSO)

http://www.surgonc.org

The Society of Surgical Oncology (SSO) is a professional association for surgical oncologists and nonphysician healthcare providers involved in oncologic patient care. On this Web site you will find information about their Annual Cancer Symposium, scientific journal, fellowship training programs, research grant opportunities, criteria for becoming a member, and much more.

The mission of the Society of Surgical Oncology is to serve its members by (1) representing and advancing the profession of surgical oncology; (2) promoting the highest quality surgical oncology patient care outcomes, education, practice, research, ethical conduct, and advocacy; and (3) promoting public policy issues related to surgical oncology.

Nurse practitioners are encouraged to attend this annual educational meeting as well as become a member of the SSO. Beginning in 2010, specific educational content will be provided that is targeted for APN professionals.

Young Survival Coalition (YSC)

155 6th Avenue, 10th Floor
New York, NY 10013
212-206-6610

info@youngsurvival.org
http://www.youngsurvival.org

The Young Survival Coalition (YSC) is the only international, nonprofit network of breast cancer survivors and supporters dedicated to the concerns and issues that are unique to young women and breast cancer. Through action, advocacy, and awareness, the YSC seeks to educate the medical, research, breast cancer, and legislative communities and to persuade them to address breast cancer in women age 40 and younger. The YSC also serves as a point of contact for young women living with breast cancer.

WHERE CAN YOUR PATIENT GET HELP WITH FINANCIAL OR LEGAL CONCERNS?

Accompanying any serious illnesses are questions and concerns related to expenses incurred as a result of treatment, health insurance questions that can be overwhelming to try and understand or resolve alone, and sometimes even legal questions related to employment or financial matters. The following is a list of national resources to aid you in addressing these types of concerns.

Cancer Care, Inc.

212-302-2400
800-813-HOPE
info@cancercare.org
http://www.cancercare.org

Cancer Care is a national, nonprofit organization that provides free, professional assistance to people with any type of cancer and to their families. This organization offers education, one-on-one counseling, financial assistance for nonmedical expenses, and referrals to community services.

Credit Counseling Centers of America (CCC America)

800-493-2222
http://www.cccamerica.org

The Credit Counseling Centers of America (CCC America) is a nonprofit organization that provides a wide array of consumer and creditor services for individuals and families experiencing financial distress.

Health Insurance Association of America

202-824-1600
800-879-4422
http://www.hiaa.org

The Health Insurance Association of America is a lobbyist group for insurance companies. They can help answer questions regarding health insurance coverage.

National Coalition for Cancer Survivorship (NCCS)

301-650-8868
877-NCCS-YES
info@ccansearch.org
http://www.cansearch.org

This network of independent groups and individuals provides information and resources about cancer support, advocacy, and quality-of-life issues as well as helping cancer patients deal with insurance or job discrimination and other related legal matters. As their name implies, they are strongly focused on improving survivorship care for all cancer patients.

Patient Advocate Foundation

757-873-6668
800-532-5274
patient@pinn.net
http://www.patientadvocate.org

This organization provides educational information about managed care/insurance issues and legal counseling on debt intervention, job discrimination issues, and denials of insurance coverage.

Social Security Administration (SSA)

Office of Public Inquiries
800-772-1213
http://www.ssa.gov

The Social Security Administration (SSA) is the U.S. government agency that runs the Social Security Program. It provides information about retirement and disability benefits, supplemental security income (SSI), and Medicare.

Together Rx Access

http://www.togetherrxaccess.com

With the free Together Rx Access Card most cardholders save 25% to 40% on more than 275 brand-name prescription drugs and other prescription products, as well as on a wide range of generic drugs. There is a list of eligible drugs on the Web site, which can be accessed from the home page. The Together Rx Access card is sponsored by some of the world's largest pharmaceutical companies, helping more people take care of their health. Those companies are Abbott Laboratories; AstraZeneca; Bristol-Myers Squibb Company; GlaxoSmithKline; Janssen Pharmaceutica Products, LP; LifeScan, a Johnson & Johnson Company; Novartis Pharmaceuticals Corporation; Ortho-McNeil Pharmaceutical, Inc.; Pfizer Inc., Sanofi-Aventis; Takeda Pharmaceuticals North America, Inc.; and TAP Pharmaceutical Products, Inc.

Index